Carb Cycling for Weight Loss for Women

Carb Cycling Made Easy with Meal Plans and Exercise Programs for Weight Loss for Beginners

RUEL FORDYCE

Copyright © 2022, Ruel Fordyce

All rights reserved.

ISBN: 9798844642562

DEDICATION

This book is dedicated to all the women who have embarked on a life-long journey to become the best version of themselves.

CONTENTS

	Quote of the Day	i
1	Could I benefit from Carb Cycling?	Pg #1
2	What does Carb Cycling Involve?	Pg #9
3	What does a Carb Cycling Diet look like?	Pg #14
4	How does Carb Cycling help with weight loss?	Pg #26
5	Are there other benefits to Carb Cycling?	Pg #30
6	What do I need to remember about Carb Cycling?	Pg #33
7	Types of Carb Cycling	Pg #39
8	Which foods are good on a Carb Cycling regime?	Pg #44
9	Sample Carb Cycling Programs	Pg #52
10	How do I get started with Carb Cycling?	Pg #61
11	Carb Cycling made easy	Pg #67
12	Home Based Training (Exercises)	Pg #84

QUOTE OF THE DAY

Some days HIGH, some days Low, some days NO!
Youri Elkaim

CHAPTER 1

COULD I BENEFIT FROM CARB CYCLING?

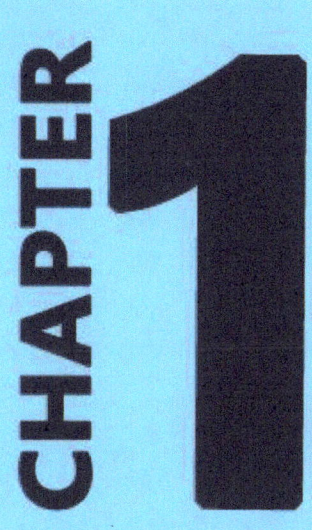

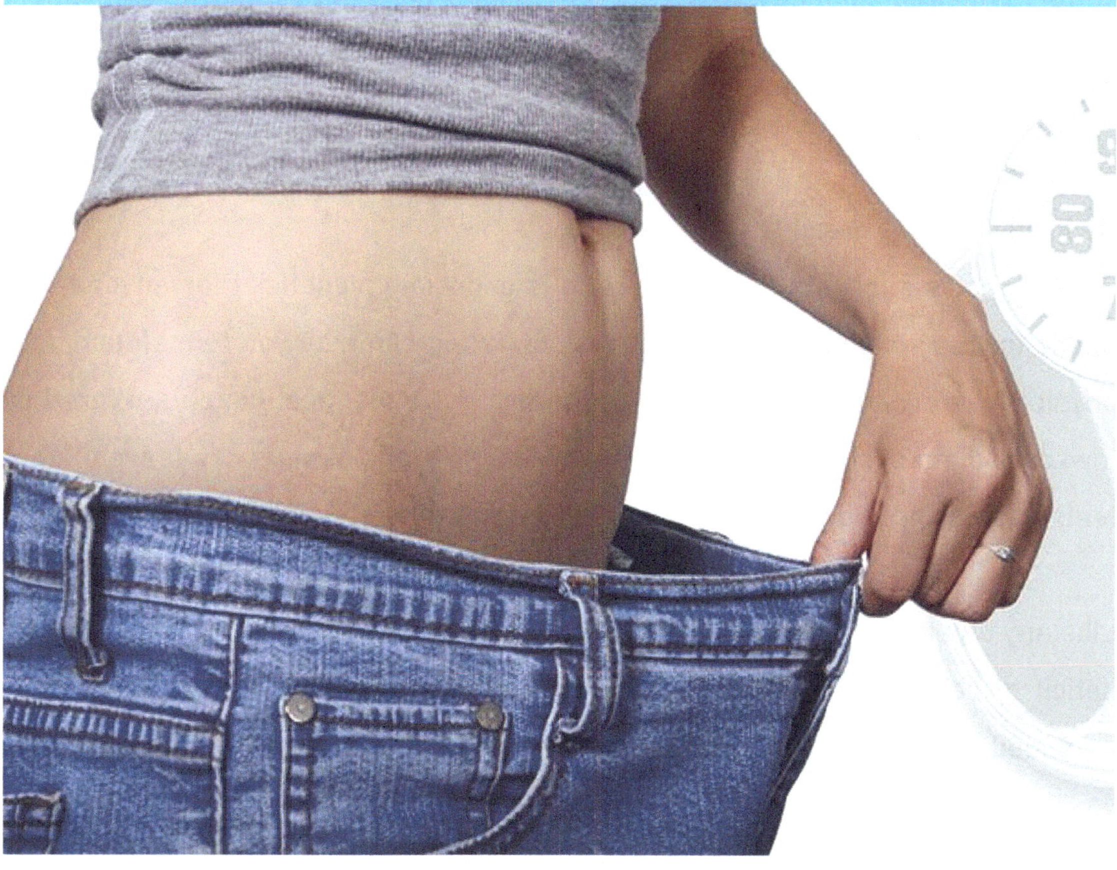

COULD I BENEFIT FROM CARB CYCLING?

Carb cycling isn't ideal for everyone. However, it can prove to be a useful solution in the right circumstances. There are two main groups of people who can benefit from trying out this eating regime: Those who need to lose weight, and those who want to increase their muscle mass while boosting their sporting performance.

Do I Need to Lose Weight?
Some experts suggest that carb cycling is especially beneficial for anyone who needs to lose weight. In theory, this way of eating can help you to maintain your physical performance. It also provides many of the identical benefits offered by low-carb diets such as the Atkins regime. These kinds of diets can leave dieters feeling lethargic and weak. Therefore, carb cycling offers a clear advantage.

Like any other diet, the primary mechanism behind losing weight is to maintain a deficit of calories. You need to eat less food than the body can burn over an extended period. When you adopt carb cycling along with a deficit in calorie intake, you'll almost certainly lose weight.

Carbohydrates aren't bad for you. However, the role of carbs is to supply an energy source for your body to burn through when you're active. If you aren't carrying out enough physical activity and are still eating a lot of carbohydrates, problems arise.

Your body ends up storing the excess as fat. Carbs are a great choice when you're working out hard in the gym. Your body will burn rapidly through them to produce energy. It burns carbs rather than protein, so this nutrient can boost muscle-growth.

If you aren't training hard, those extra carbs aren't being burned up quickly. Therefore, the body stores all the unused glucose in the fat cells. This results in you becoming overweight or even obese.

On the other hand, if you restrict carb intake, your body cannot store the excess glucose. Instead, it turns to fats to produce energy rather than starchy or sugary foods. As a result, your body can shed fat, helping you lose weight.

Hoarding additional calories is all well and good if you have a very active lifestyle. Yet, if you aren't moving around much, you cannot use all those calories. This leads to obesity. You therefore need to vary your carb intake from day to day. If you're going to be hitting the gym, you can eat more carbs. If you're going to be watching TV for most of the day, you should restrict your intake.

Another reason why carb cycling is so good for weight loss is because it makes it hard to overeat. Foods with a high carb count are usually more indulgent. We all know how hard it is to resist the urge to eat another cookie or a delicious, sugary donut. It's a lot harder to binge eat on vegetables and proteins. Very few people will over-indulge on chicken or broccoli! Therefore, you'll be consuming fewer calories and helping your waistline.

As carb cycling is a flexible way to diet, it can be more appealing to dieters. Knowing that you can indulge in carbs occasionally can be attractive. One of the reasons why so many people fail with other diets is because of their restrictive nature.

Knowing you can never eat pasta or bread can be off-putting from the start. This leads to dieters giving up after a short while. Carb cycling's flexibility can encourage these people to adhere to the program. As a result, they'll lose more weight overall and maintain a healthier bodyweight.

There is also a key link between levels of insulin in the blood and carb intake. If there is a high level of insulin in the blood, fat storage becomes more likely. In turn, this hinders effective weight loss. You should take care about changing your carb intake if you're taking insulin for diabetes. Therefore, talking to a doctor is key.

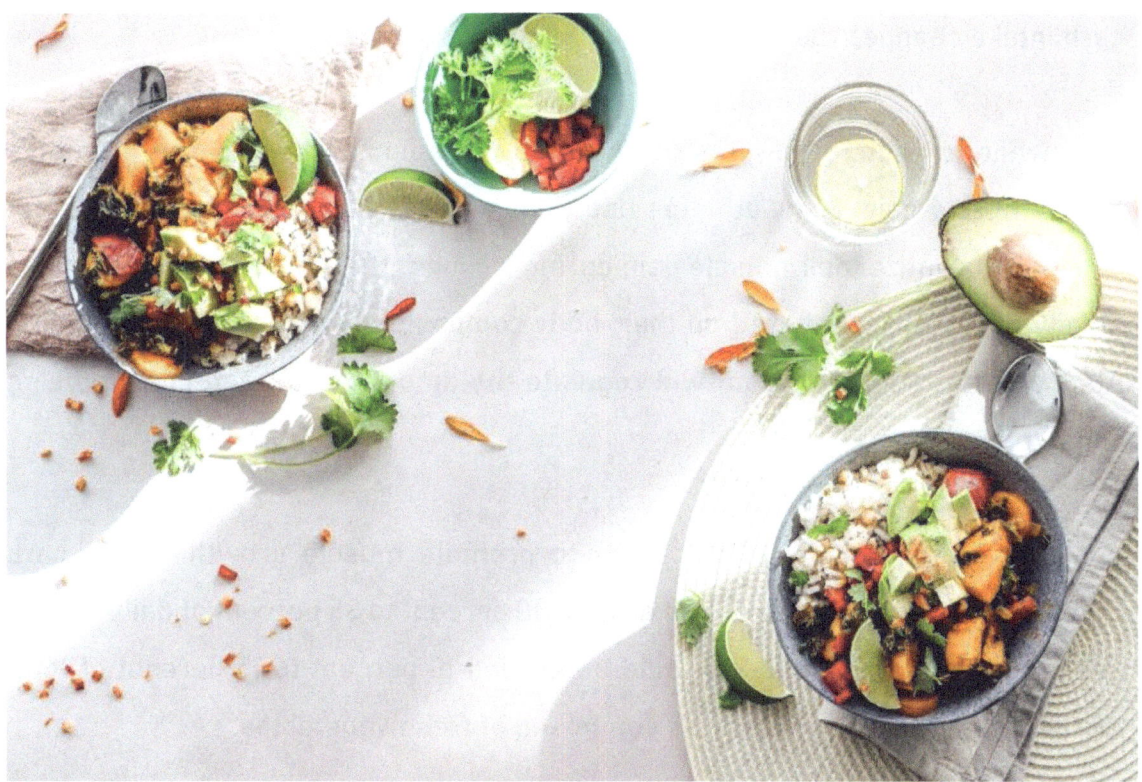

Healthy eating must also lie at the heart of any carb cycling plan. It isn't an excuse to restrict eating to excess or over-indulge on unhealthy food. Meticulous tracking is required to be successful at carb cycling. This can promote an unhealthy attitude towards eating. Therefore, you need to take care to stay in perspective when adopting this regime. If you find it's negatively affecting your life in this way, you should stop and choose a different eating plan.

Am I a Bodybuilder?

Carb cycling remains a popular strategy for nutrition for athletes and bodybuilders. Those who are physique competitors are especially keen on this way of eating. They depend heavily on no or low carb days in their competition preparation cutting phase. Since glycogen is primarily water, manipulating your carb intake changes the appearance of muscles onstage.

Meanwhile, creating a surplus of energy by consuming more carbs promotes better muscle gain. Many athletes use their way of eating to minimize their fat gain and maximize their muscle gain during training. They must strictly adhere to a daily menu which is based on their body composition and energy expenditure. Also, a carb cycling program will regulate the amount of fat and protein being consumed.

A higher protein intake is necessary to promote muscle growth during carb cycling. Protein must therefore be around 30 percent to 35 percent of daily calorie intake. Carbs in a low phase should be around 10 percent to 15 percent of total intake. These should primarily be composed of fresh vegetables.

High carb days should fall on days of intense training. This will ensure muscle recovery is faster and essential nutrients are provided. By having targeted carb intakes and regular periods of high carbs, your performance can improve. For athletes participating in endurance sports such as swimming, cycling, and running, this is good news. Varying carb intake through the year helps to increase stores of muscle glycogen.

Carb cycling optimizes the carb load so there's enough fuel to burn when working out intensively. Nevertheless, excess carbs won't be stored as far when you're having a non-workout day. Elite athletes have been eating this way for some time. They believe it helps them to boost their workout performance.

At the same time, they can build muscle while maintaining a healthy bodyweight. Bodybuilders and athletes who carb cycle also have shorter recovery times. Their glycogen replenishment gets a boost and nutrients are delivered more effectively. As a result, they can enjoy better gains in the gym.

Is Carb Cycling Suitable for Everyone?

Unfortunately, carb cycling isn't the answer for everyone. In theory, it should be a suitable way of eating for anyone. However, some people fail to carry it out properly. This could cause health problems and ongoing issues. When you follow any restrictive diet, you need to be aware of when it's time to stop.

If you constantly crave foods which are "off limits" and feel guilty if you indulge, this is a red flag. Also, if you find that carb cycling is negatively affecting your attitude and mood, this could be a problem. It's a sign that this way of eating isn't for you.

Also, if you're unusually fatigued when carb cycling, this is a sign to stop. Anyone who has a history of eating disorders should avoid carb cycling. Restriction and adherence together with measuring, tracking, and counting are key elements of this diet. Constantly being aware of carb and calorie intake reinforces disordered eating patterns. This can worsen eating disorders and cause new issues to develop.

People who have certain medical conditions should avoid carb cycling. People who have mood disorders like depression and anxiety may be adversely affected. Changing eating patterns can lead to worse mood swings which worsen mental health problems.

People suffering from other medical conditions like heart disease and metabolic syndrome should also be wary. This also applies to those suffering from diabetes. Although carb cycling can be good for regulating insulin levels, it can be problematic for those on medication. If you're taking insulin for diabetes already, you must talk to your doctor before trying this diet.

Failing to do this could lead to damaging results for your overall health and wellbeing. Some other people should also avoid carb cycling. Women who are pregnant, for example, should avoid any diet of this type. They need to have a steady ongoing supply of carbohydrates that are rich in fiber to remain healthy. For the same reason, breastfeeding mothers should also steer clear of this dietary regime.

However, when carb cycling is followed properly, it should be a suitable way of eating for everyone. Many dieters find the flexibility of this regime suits their preferences. They can still enjoy carbs occasionally and this makes them feel less restricted. They also often find that the monotony of a regular diet is reduced. It's therefore often recommended that you consult your doctor before trying carb cycling. A medical professional will be able to suggest whether it's a good choice for you.

CHAPTER 2

WHAT DOES CARB CYCLING INVOLVE?

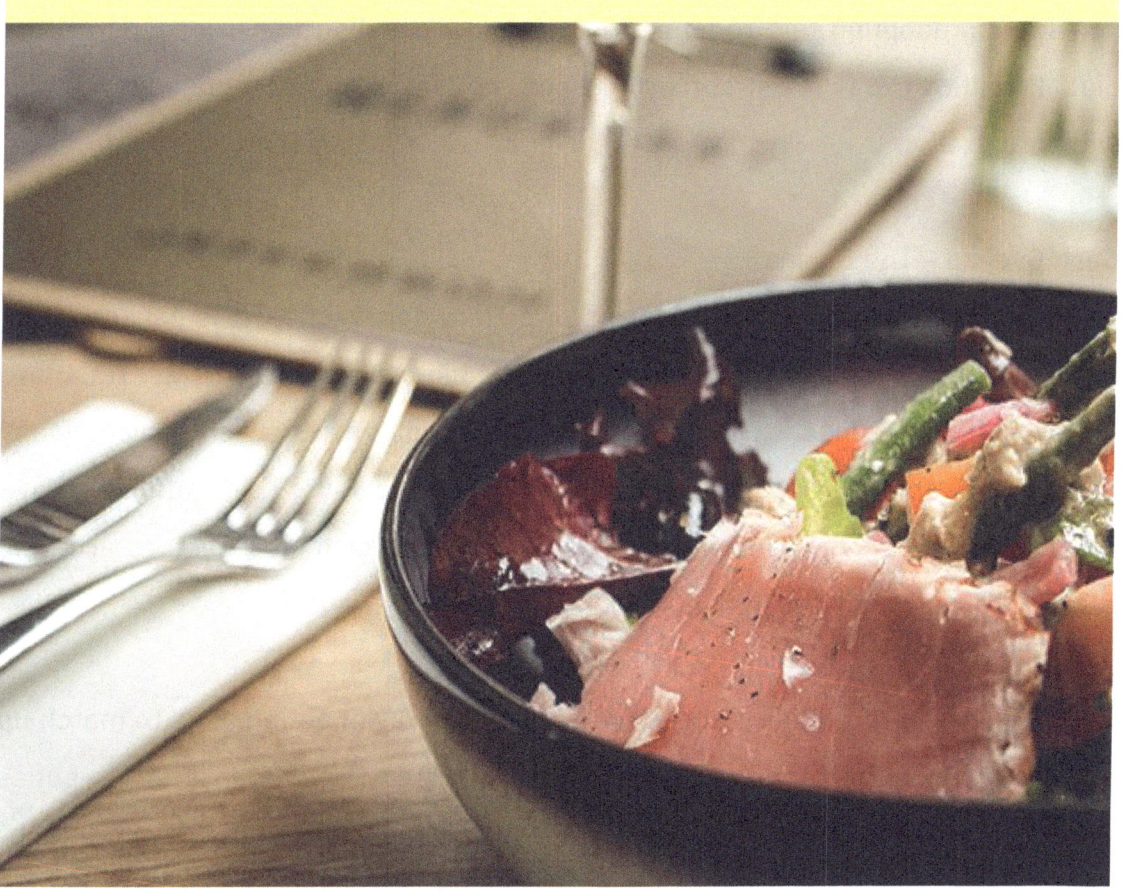

WHAT DOES CARB CYCLING INVOLVE?

Knowing the science behind why carb cycling works is important for anyone considering adopting this regime. Without understanding the principles of this diet, it's difficult to follow it correctly. Here, we look at the basics so you can be well informed.

Carb Cycling – The Basics
Carb cycling is relatively new in terms of dietary approaches. It is backed up by science based on carbohydrate manipulation's biological mechanisms. Yet, there are few official studies which have directly investigated carb cycling diets. Many people have found this regime a successful one, however. Elite athletes have been using this method for years to boost their performance. Dieters are also starting to recognize the benefits.

So, how does carb cycling work? Essentially, this way of eating aims to match up the body's requirement for glucose or calories. For instance, it supplies carbohydrates on days of intense training or workouts. It achieves this by planning in days of high carbohydrate intake on those days. High carbohydrate days refuel glycogen in the muscles. This too can reduce breakdown of the muscles and improve sporting performance.

When high-carbohydrate periods are strategically planned, it's possible to boost the functioning of appetite-regulating hormones. Ghrelin and leptin are both hormones associated with hunger and appetite. Both can be better controlled with carb cycling diets.

On low carbohydrate days, the body switches to a different way of producing energy. Without the glucose from carbs to fuel it, it predominantly begins to burn fat. This, in turn, helps to improve the body's metabolic flexibility. It also helps the body to adapt more effectively to burning fat as a fuel source over the long-term.

Another major element in carb cycling is how it allows insulin to be manipulated. If you target your carbs around your workouts, it can improve your body's sensitivity to insulin. This is a sign of good health. It helps to protect against conditions like diabetes. It also helps to maximize the many benefits that carbohydrates provide.

Is Carb Cycling the Same as Keto?
Many people think that the keto diet and carb cycling are the same things. This isn't true. Although there are some similarities, the two regimes are very different. The keto diet is extremely low in carbohydrates. It also involves eating a lot of good fats and moderate amounts of protein. The main aim of the keto diet is to burn fat as fuel by getting into ketosis.

Usually, carb cycling involves eating more carbs than you would have in the classic keto diet. It also doesn't involve eating the same large amount of fats. Therefore, ketosis isn't the aim of a carb cycling regime. Nevertheless, there are some similarities. Both emphasize the management of carbohydrate intake. Also, both diets involve counting macros. Macros are the specific number of grams of fats, protein and carbs you eat every day. This means that some people combine both regimes. This is known as keto cycling.

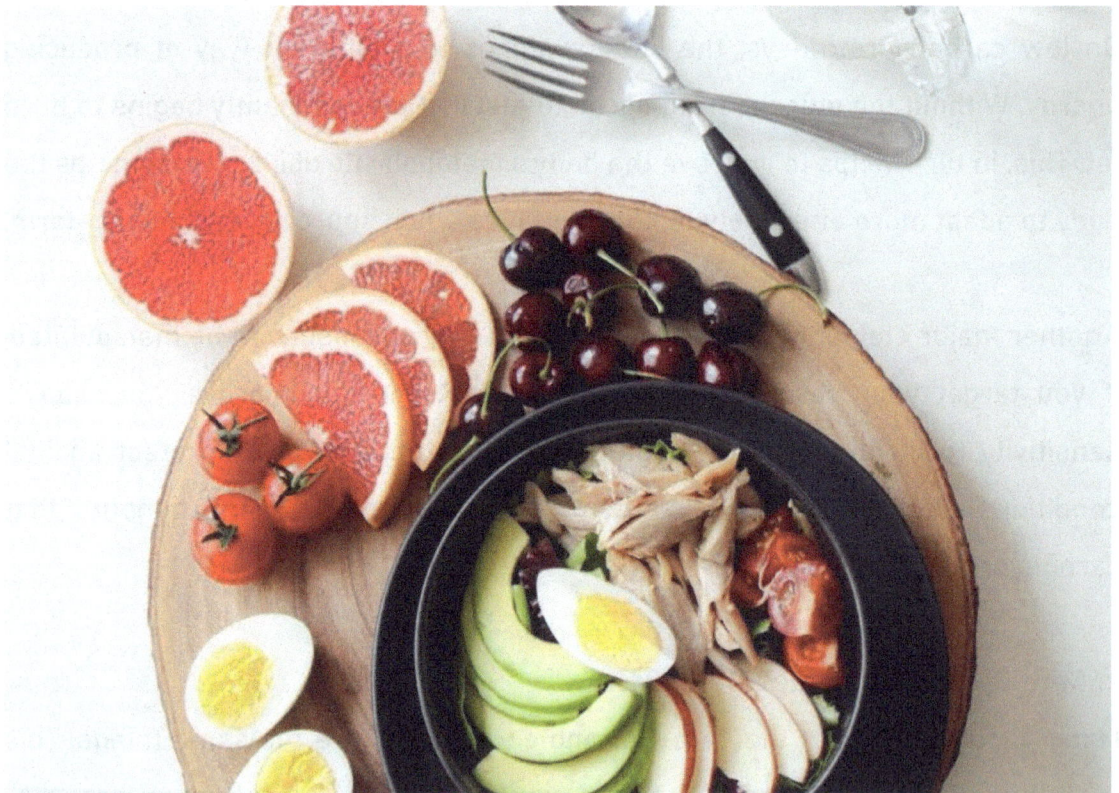

The keto cycling protocol involves eating a keto diet on most days. These will be interspersed with either one or two days of eating more carbs. These are called re-feeding days. They are designed to break the ketosis. By doing this, dieters can receive the benefits of consuming carbohydrates. Their fiber intake is increased, their athletic performance is fueled, and their diet is more varied. Some nutritional experts say that restricting carbs in the long-term could impact on certain hormones. Insulin and thyroid hormones are vital for healthy body composition.

If you try keto-cycling, balance in these hormones could be better maintained. This provides a distinct advantage over the standard keto diet in which carbs are restricted over an extended period. Not only that, but the common problems associated with keto diets are reduced or eliminated. Issues such as bad breath don't become prevalent since some carbs are still being consumed regularly.

CHAPTER 3
WHAT DOES A CARB CYCLING DIET LOOK LIKE?

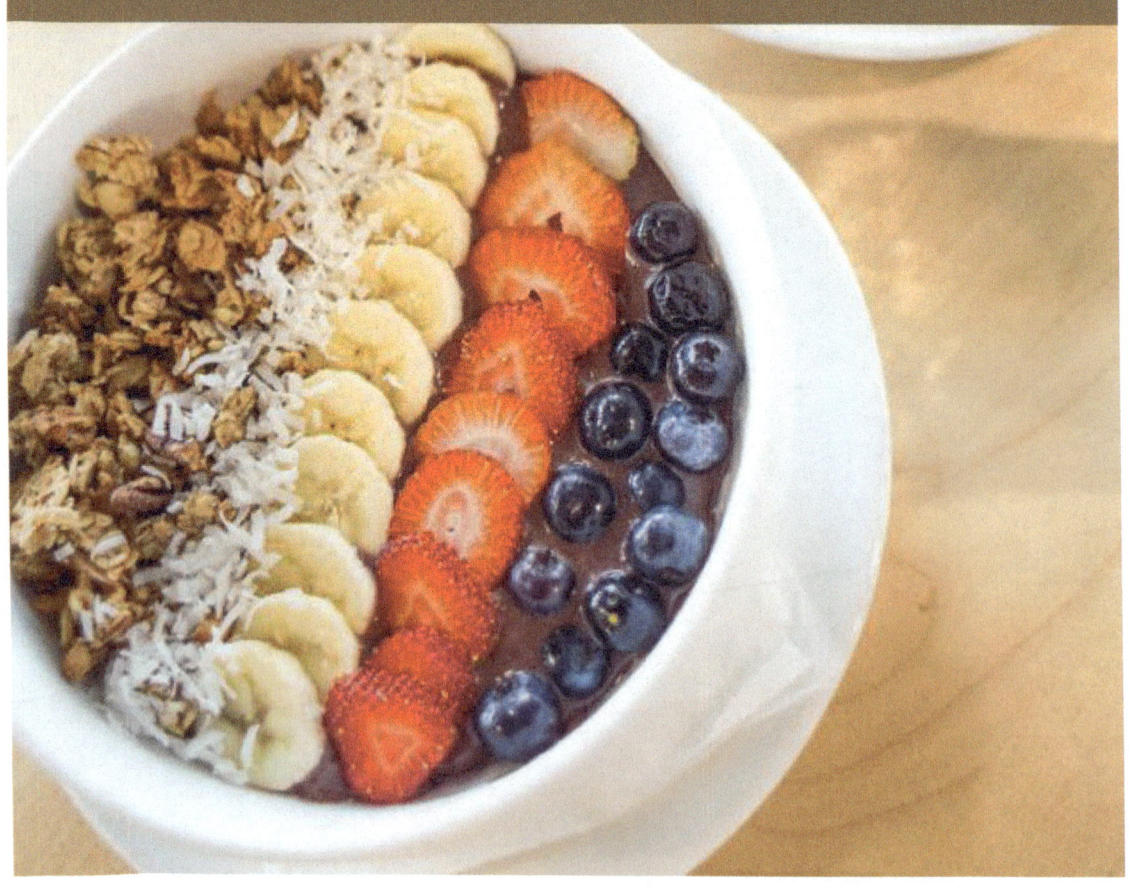

WHAT DOES A CARB CYCLING DIET LOOK LIKE?

Carb cycling involves tracking macros with a food journal or app. You must work out the number of grams of carbohydrates you'll need to eat every day. This may not be as easy as you imagined. The amount of carbs you should eat will be individual to you. You need to bear several factors in mind. We'll look more closely at those later. For now, let's take a closer look at what a standard carb cycling diet looks like.

What do I eat on a High Carb Day?
On a high carb day, you will usually obtain around 60 percent of your calories from complex carbohydrates. That means if you're eating about 1,500 calories daily, around 900 calories are complex carbs.

If you're doing high energy workouts like interval training, long distance running or sprints, you can add in more carbs. These should take the right form though. You shouldn't be adding donuts or cake into your regime! Instead, you should give yourself an additional serving of legumes, fruits, or whole grains. The latter are all complex carbs. This means they break down more slowly for a slower release of energy.

Simple carbs like sugary cookies and candies break down quickly. This means that you get a super-fast energy rush followed by a crash. You should primarily eat complex carbohydrates on a carb cycling regime. If you find that you're struggling to cope with your athletic workouts, try adding another serving into your diet. You should only do this on days when you're hitting the gym though.

What Do I Eat On A Low Carb Day?
On days when you're not working out or doing low-key exercise, have a low carb day. On this kind of day, you should switch a couple of your usual carb servings with vegetables. You could also switch some of those carbs with healthy fats or proteins.

Alternatively, you could use a low-carb day as a starting point from which to calculate your high carb days. Usually, 50 grams of carbs daily is enough to reach ketosis. Therefore, you could begin by consuming 50 grams of carbs on low carb days. You can then work up from there, maxing out at 200 grams of carbs daily. Avoiding the transactional food mindset is very important, however.

Thoughts like "30 minutes more running means I can eat more carbs" can be dangerous. It leads to a difficult and disordered relationship with eating and food. Nevertheless, eating more carbs some days with fewer carbs on other days is how the body regulates itself naturally. Therefore, reducing carbs offers benefits that you can take advantage of.

What Does A Week-Long Carb Cycling Plan Look Like?

The concept of carb cycling involves eating minimal carbs for two days consecutively. This will be followed by a day of eating more carbs. There is a reason for this. When the stored reserves of carbs are due to run out, energy is recharged thanks to a high carb day. This speeds the metabolism and leads to more fat loss.

If you reduce your carbs over two days, your fat stores will be used for energy. Your body will also enter a catabolic state. This means the body starts to use muscle tissue to derive energy from the protein in your muscles. It's important to know what to eat over a week if you're planning to carb cycle. Here is a sample seven-day plan to ensure you obtain all the essential nutrients. You'll also get enough variety, so you don't get bored with your meals. If you can adhere to this plan for 30 days, you should experience weight loss benefits.

Day 1 - A Low Carb Day

Breakfast: Almond and citrus fruit salad mixed with berries and yogurt.

Snack: An apple and a protein bar.

Lunch: Salad made with 50 grams of quinoa, 100 grams of peas and tomatoes and two hard-boiled eggs.

Snack: A banana and a scoop of walnuts.

Dinner: A sliced stir-fried chicken breast with sliced carrots, courgettes, and green beans. Served with 70 grams of quinoa.

Snack: Two oatcakes.

Calorie Total - 1880
Carbs Total - 226 grams
Protein Total - 108 grams
Fat Total - 67 grams

Day 2 – Low Carb Day

Breakfast: Seed and apple muesli made with two tablespoons of rolled oats, sunflower seeds, sesame seeds and pumpkin seeds. Served with two tablespoons of natural yogurt and a small apple.

Snack: A banana and scoop of walnuts.

Lunch: A whole meal pitta stuffed with half an avocado, one tablespoon of cottage cheese and tuna.

Snack: A pear.

Dinner: A grilled salmon steak with half a sliced lime on top. Served with 100 grams broccoli, 70 grams of quinoa and 75 grams of peas.

Snack: An apple.

Calorie Total – 1891
Carbs Total – 170 grams
Protein Total – 131 grams
Fat Total – 81 grams

Day 3 – High Carb Day

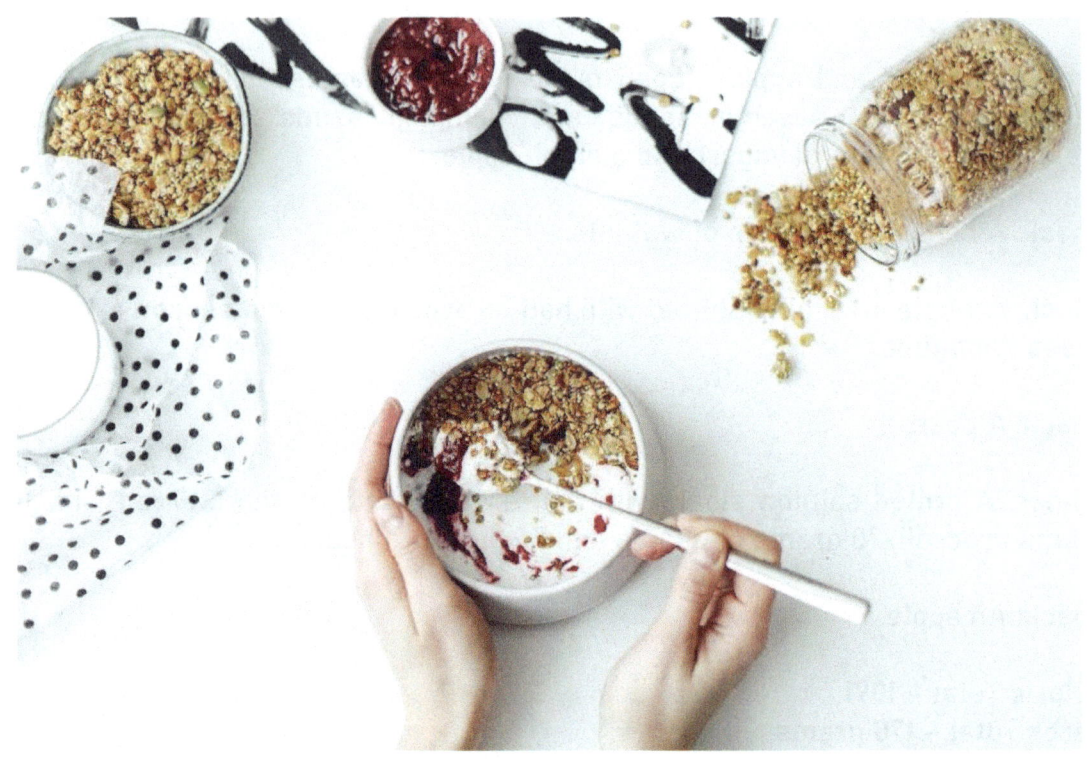

Breakfast: 60 grams of oats, soaked in water with 200 grams of berries. Serve with a pot of natural yogurt and a tablespoon of sunflower seeds.

Snack: A peach.

Lunch: A baked potato stuffed with a tablespoon of hummus. Serve with salad made from sliced cucumber, tomato, red pepper, and mixed leaves. A banana.

Snack: A protein bar and an apple.

Dinner: A grilled cod fillet served with 250 grams of boiled potatoes, 100 grams of carrots and peas.

Snack: Three oatcakes.

Calorie Total – 1801
Carbs Total – 323 grams
Protein Total – 78 grams
Fat Total – 40 grams

Day 4 – Low Carb Day

Breakfast: three eggs beaten with two tablespoons of natural yogurt. Add half a red pepper, half a courgette and half an onion as well as one tablespoon of peas. Cook in a pan.

Snack: An apple and a handful of pumpkin seeds.

Lunch: A can of salmon mixed with a can of butter beans. Serve with a salad of lettuce leaves, tomato, sugar snap peas, and onion.

Snack: A nectarine.

Dinner: A grilled turkey breast with grilled courgette, carrot, red pepper, and onion.

Snack: A banana and 80 grams of grapes.

Calorie Total – 1812
Carbs Total – 159 grams
Protein Total – 143 grams
Fat Total – 72 grams

Day 5 – Low Carb Day

Breakfast: Two boiled eggs with two whole meal pitta slices spread with Marmite and butter.

Snack: An apple and a pear.

Lunch: Avocado and tuna mash served with salad leaves, cucumber, tomato, carrot, and courgette.

Snack: A peace and an oatcake topped with cucumber and cottage cheese.

Dinner: A can of salmon mixed with a can of chopped tomatoes, tomato puree, carrot, red pepper, and courgettes. Simmered for 10 minutes and served.

Snack: A banana.

Calorie Total – 1804
Carbs Total – 165 grams
Protein Total – 124 grams
Fat Total – 77 grams

Day 6 – High Carb Day

Breakfast: 5 tablespoons of natural yogurt. Mix with 50 grams of rolled oats, 200 grams of berries, 1 tablespoon of honey and a sliced pear.

Snack: A whole meal pitta bread stuffed with a tomato and cottage cheese.

Lunch: A chickpea salad made with half a can of chickpeas.

Snack: Four oatcakes with sliced apple and peanut butter.

Dinner: A grilled chicken breast with steamed broccoli, 70g quinoa and 100g green beans.

Snack: A banana.

Calorie Total – 1845
Carbs Total – 249 grams
Protein Total – 122 grams
Fat Total – 44 grams

Day 7 – Low Carb Day

Breakfast: Two poached eggs with two portobello mushrooms and two tomatoes.

Snack: A pot of natural yogurt, an orange, and a peach.

Lunch: A pitta stuffed with cottage cheese, avocado, cucumber, tomato, lettuce, and peanut butter.

Snack: An apple with a handful of sunflower seeds and pumpkin seeds.

Dinner: Poached salmon with a courgette, 200 grams tomatoes and sugar snap peas.

Snack: A banana and two oatcakes.

Calorie Total – 1820
Carbs Total – 157 grams
Protein Total – 98 grams
Fat Total – 94 grams

CHAPTER 4
HOW DOES CARB CYCLING HELP WITH WEIGHT LOSS?

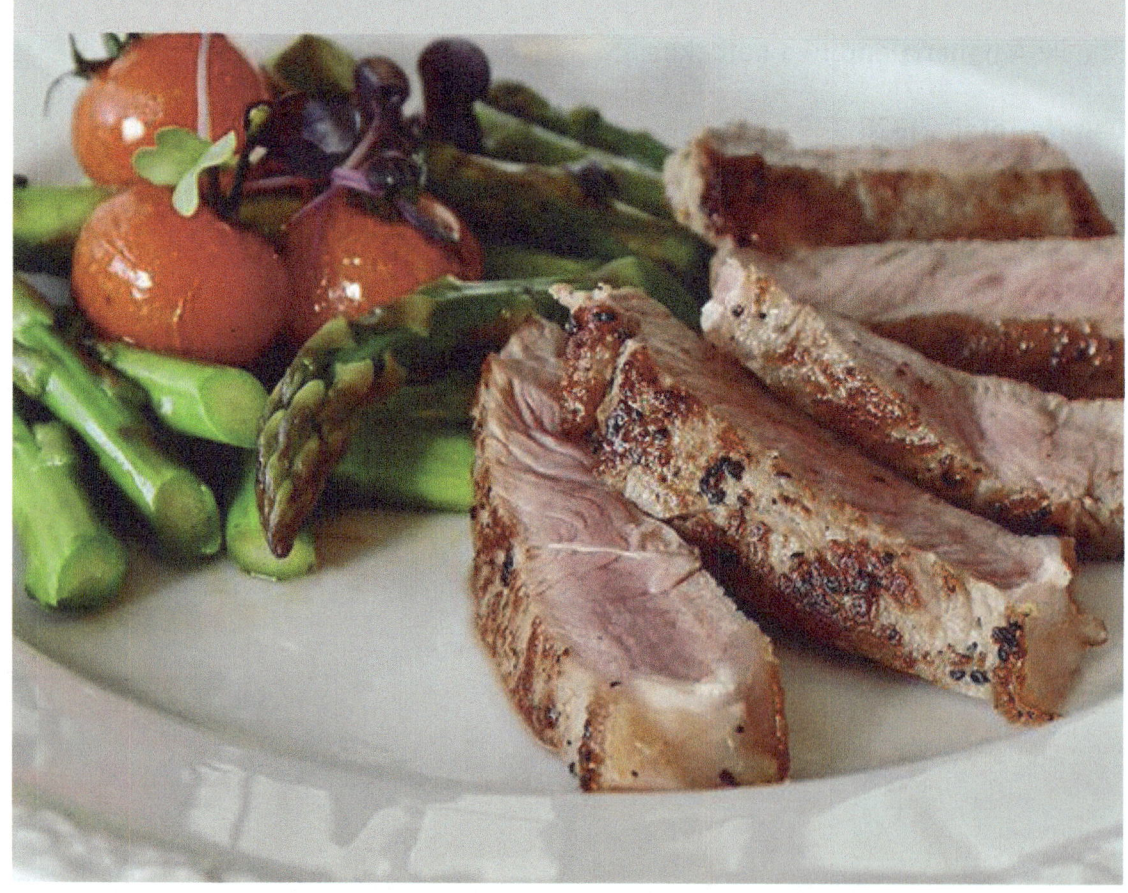

HOW DOES CARB CYCLING HELP WITH WEIGHT LOSS?

Carb cycling can help with weight loss by maximizing how the body uses fuel. When you adopt this diet, you eat fewer carbs for two days then have a day of eating more carbs. How you alternate between high and low carb days varies depending on how much activity you're doing. You benefit from the carb fuel you get on the days when you're working out. Meanwhile, you benefit from low carbs if you're not active.

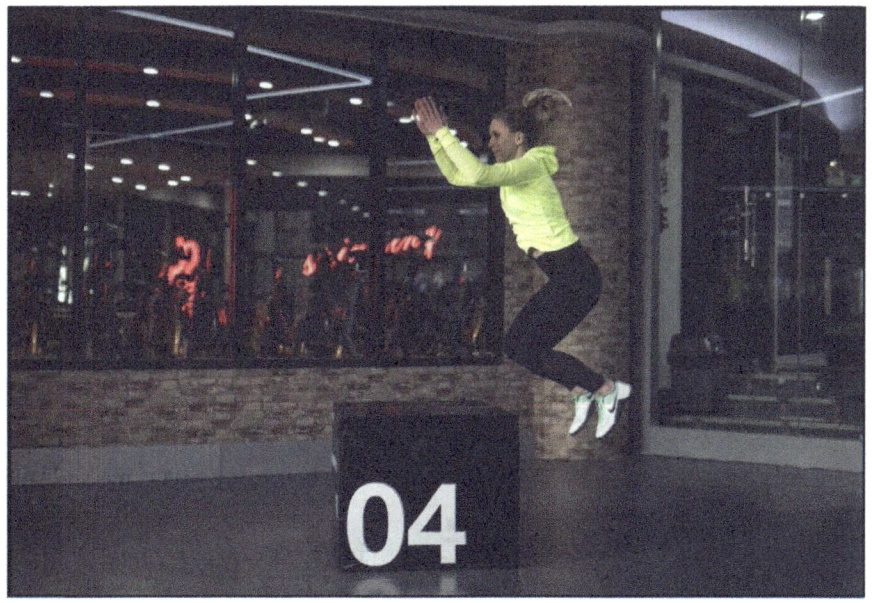

As you work out, the body dips into its carbohydrate stores to find energy. This means you should align high carb days with training days. This means your body can use the fuel to its best advantage. It also means that the additional energy allows you to work out for longer. You'll therefore burn more calories as a result. On rest days, carbs can be scaled back. This will reduce the number of empty calories you consume and help you lose weight.

Imagine your weight is 175 pounds. You could aim to have two grams of carbs for every pound of your weight on a high carb day. That would be around 350 grams. On low carb days, you could reduce this to around one gram per pound of your weight. This would take your carb intake down to 175 grams. That doesn't mean there's a set amount of carbs you can eat on each type of day. Largely, it depends on what workout you're doing. It also depends on how frequently you're working out.

You'll find plenty of advice online. However, you'll need to tailor your carbohydrate intake to your own needs. Your metabolism will decrease or increase depending on your macronutrient and calorie intake. If you eat enough carbs at the correct time, your metabolism is reset. This triggers your body to release leptin and thyroid. These are hormones which regulate your body weight.

The SAD (Standard American Diet) is very heavy in carbs. This can produce a negative effect, stimulating the release of insulin too often. As a result, weight gain can occur and conditions like diabetes can develop. Low carb days encourage your body to use all its glycogen (stored carbs). It switches to burning ketones (body fat) as fuel. When stored fat is burned, weight is naturally lost. Every carb cycling diet plan is different. You need to choose the one that meets your own goals. A standard plan will keep your carb intake very low for two to three days. It will then increase your carb intake for a day. That day should involve some intense activity.

On a low carb take, your carbohydrate intake should be around 50 grams to 150 grams. It should come from dairy and non-starchy vegetables. On a high carb day, you can have around 400 grams of carbs. These can come from starchy carbs, fruit, and wholegrains as well as dairy and non-starchy vegetables.

CHAPTER 5
ARE THERE OTHER BENEFITS TO CARB CYCLING?

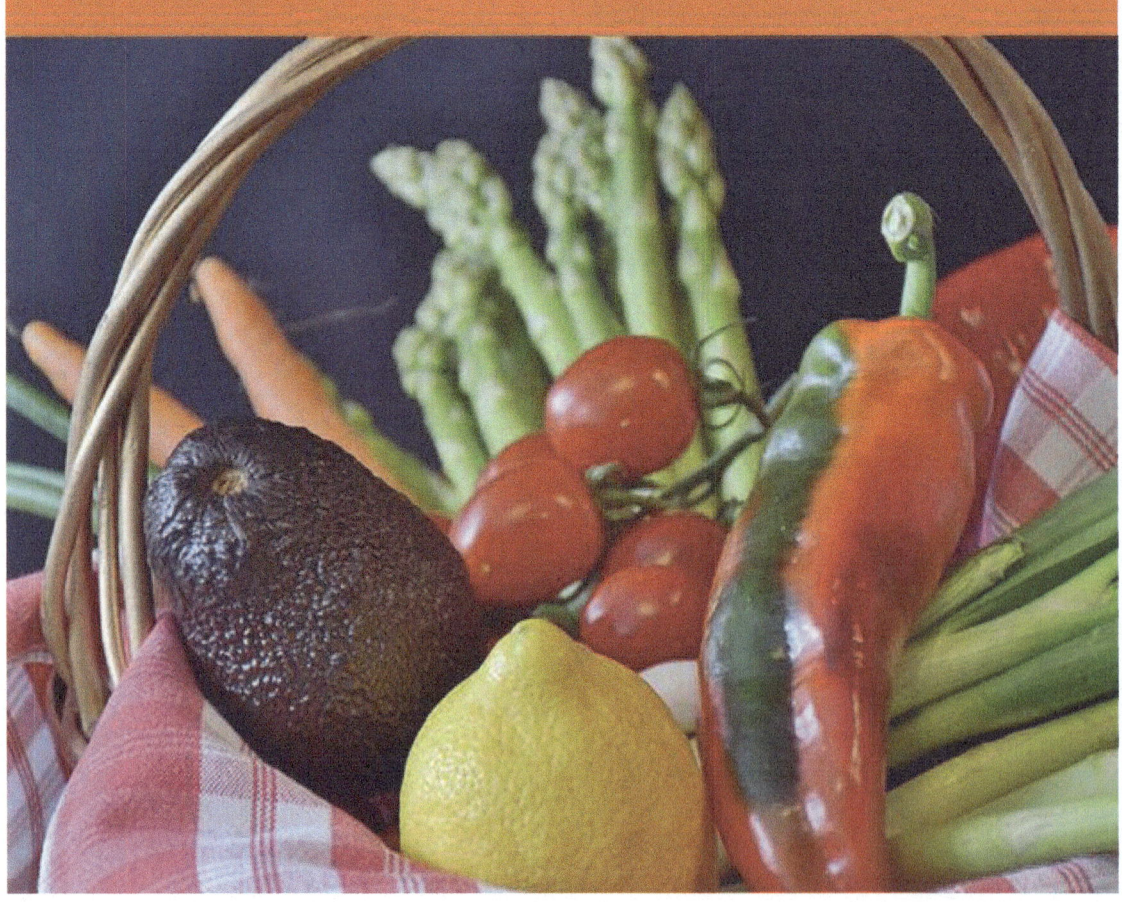

ARE THERE OTHER BENEFITS TO CARB CYCLING?

Carb cycling's primary benefit is rapid weight loss. However, there are some other benefits offered by this way of eating that other diets don't provide. When you cycle between high and low carb days, you reap the benefits offered by both forms of dieting.

Even better, many of the negatives of those diets are eliminated. Some of the benefits of carb cycling include improved insulin sensitivity. This helps to reduce the risk of developing type 2 diabetes. It can also improve cholesterol levels and enhance metabolic health. Anyone who is pre-diabetic, insulin resistant, or who has type 2 diabetes already can benefit from this way of eating.

Also, those who are resistant to weight loss may benefit from this regime. By decreasing carb intake, insulin release is also reduced. This allows the body to burn rapidly through carbohydrate stores, switching to burning fat for energy instead. As a result, faster weight loss can be triggered.

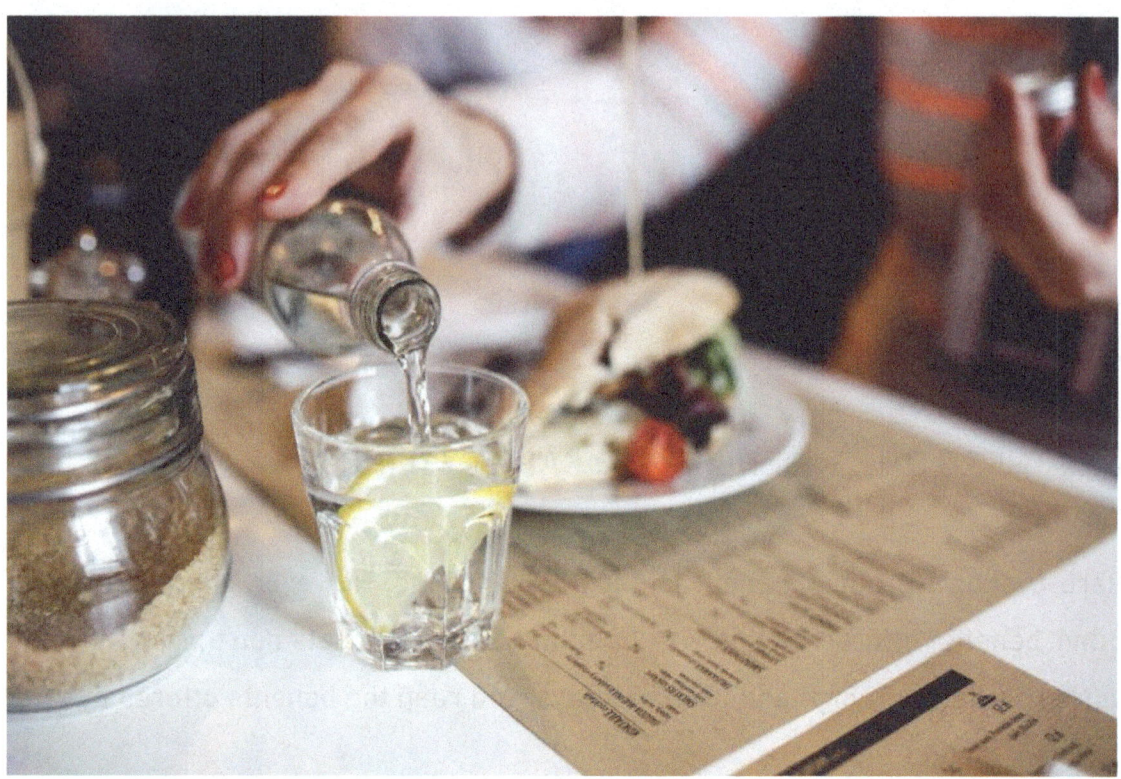

During the higher carb refeeding period, hormones can enjoy positive effects. Thyroid hormones, leptin and testosterone can all reap a positive impact. All these factors have a key role to play in dieting success over the long-term. Hormones play a vital part in exercise performance, metabolism, and hunger management. Therefore, controlling them more efficiently will ensure better function.

CHAPTER 6

WHAT DO I NEED TO REMEMBER ABOUT CARB CYCLING?

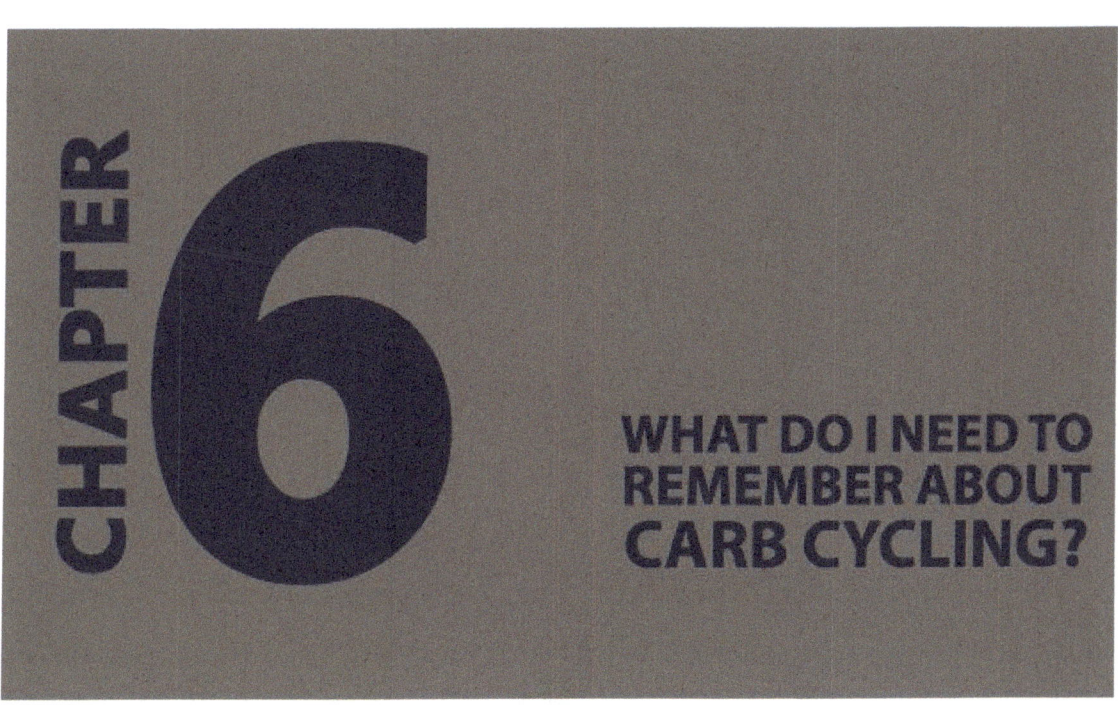

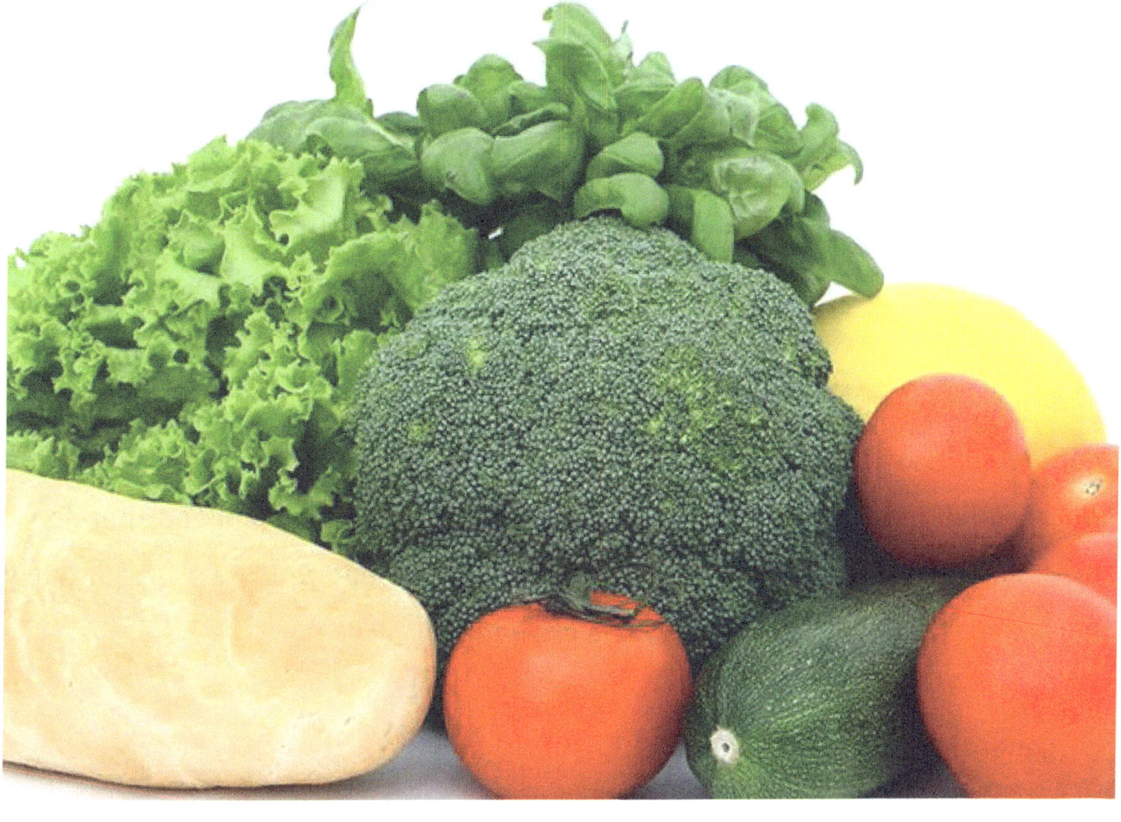

WHAT DO I NEED TO REMEMBER ABOUT CARB CYCLING?

Carb cycling isn't an effort-free way of eating. Many people embark on this regime without realizing how much work is involved. Planning is key to your success. You need to measure, count grams and weigh to be able to succeed. There are apps out there such as My Fitness Pal which can make life easier. However, if you want a regime that is all planned out for you carb cycling isn't for you. On the other hand, if rules and guidelines are your preferred option, carb cycling is a great choice. Are you thinking about giving it a try? Then read on to find out what you must remember about this way of eating.

Get it Right for You
Your first step is to make sure you get your carb cycling regime right for you as an individual. Everyone has different carb intake needs. That means there's no single one size fits all solution. You'll need to work out your own unique daily calorie goal for each day. This can be a challenge.

One general approach to take is:

- Want to lose weight? Multiply your weight by ten. This is the number of calories you should aim to consume each day.
- Want to maintain your existing weight? Multiply your weight by 12. This is the number of calories you'll need to eat daily.
- Want to gain weight? Multiply your weight by 15. This is how many calories you'll need to eat daily.

Once you know the number of calories to aim for, it's time to move on to the next step. You need to divide up those calories amongst the three main macronutrients: fat, protein and carbohydrates. Protein and carbs both supply four calories per gram. Fat provides nine calories per gram. As well as carb cycling, you should aim for around one gram of protein for each pound of your weight. The rest should be made up of healthy fats.

On a high carb day, you'll increase the number of carbs you eat. You'll also increase your calorie intake. The fats and protein levels will remain the same. On low carb days, you'll reduce your calorie intake. Again, your fat and protein levels will remain the same. Essentially, carb cycling is about reducing your calorie intake, but not feeling as if you are.

It's important to remember that if you keep your carbs too low for several days you can experience ill-effects. Carb cravings, fatigue, sleep problems, bloating, irritability, moodiness, and constipation can all occur as a result. This happens because your body has used up all its available carbohydrates and is switching to using fat as fuel. It's a phenomenon known as "carb flu". It is temporary but if you maintain your hydration level and consume enough electrolytes it'll pass quickly.

Not everyone can cope with carb cycling regimes, though. For some people, it's a counter-productive way to eat. People suffering from Hashimoto's Disease or who have adrenal fatigue can find their thyroid hormone production is reduced. This can slow down their metabolic rate and cause weight gain. People who are breastfeeding, pregnant, have a history of eating disorders or who are already underweight should avoid this regime.

Calories and Protein
When you're carb cycling, it can be tempting to eradicate lots of things from your diet. It's important to remember that it's only refined carbs that need to be slashed. When you're eating fewer carbs, you need to ensure that fiber remains a key part of your diet. A low carb day isn't a reason to forget apples or broccoli. Primarily, focus on taking out simple carbs and sugar from your diet. Bagels and muffins can go.

Nutrient-rich, fiber-filled foods like quinoa, oats, beans, fruits, and vegetables should all stay. If you prioritize high-fiber carbohydrates on your low carb days, you'll feel fuller. Your cholesterol levels will be better controlled, and your microbiome will be healthier. This will help you to manage your weight effectively since you won't be tempted to binge. Inflammation will also be reduced, helping to combat obesity.

You may think you can lose more weight if you reduce your calorie intake significantly. However, you still need to eat enough. Even on a low carb day, you need to maintain appropriate calorie intake.

The brain requires carbohydrates to function. Specifically, it requires glucose to run effectively. If there is no glucose for it to use, the body must use another source. It may end up using protein for this purpose. This is bad news when you want to maintain and build up lean muscle. You must, therefore, eat over 130 grams of carbs even on a low carb day. The brain needs to be fed so you don't spend the whole day walking around in a fog.

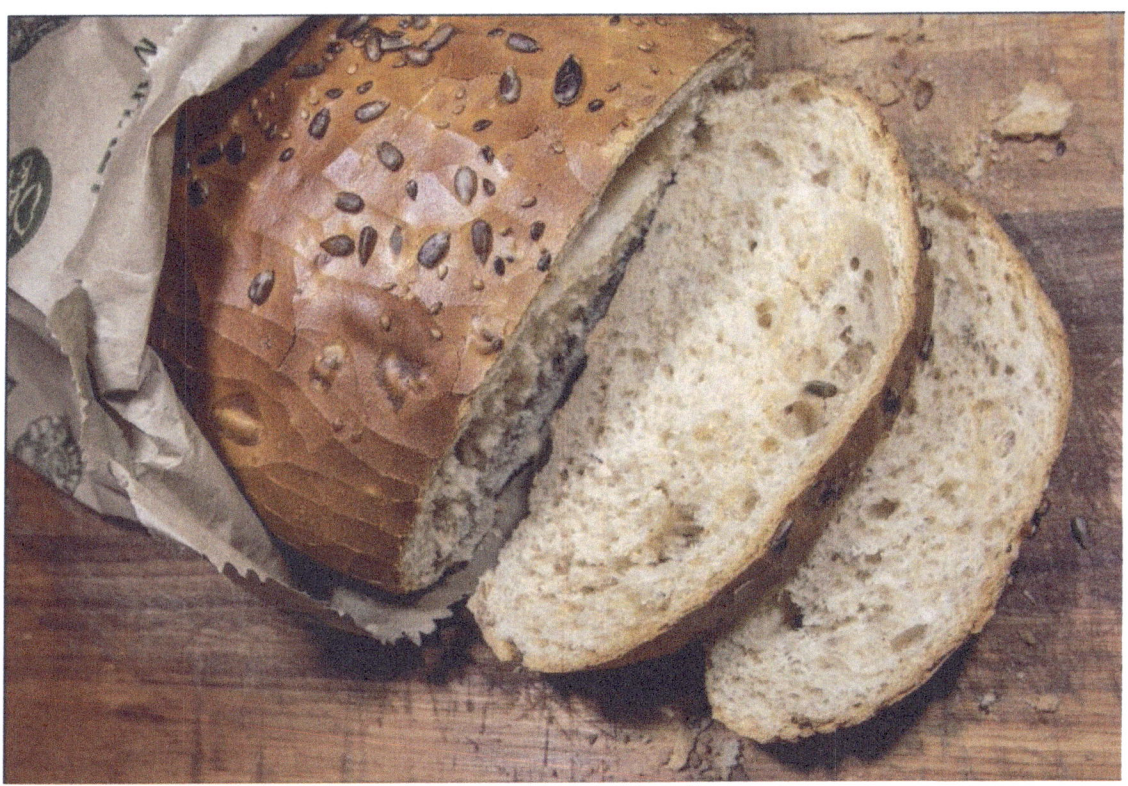

Remember that the quality of the food you eat matters just as much as the amount. Your high carbohydrate days mustn't be filled with fries and pizza! You should enjoy whole grains instead. Wholegrain pasta and bread and brown rice are much healthier options than refined sugars.

If you aren't sure what you should be eating, you should talk to an expert. The amount of carbs that you'll need will vary depending on your make-up. It will vary depending on your calorific needs, your activity level, and the type of exercise you do.

It'll also vary depending on your height, weight, and gender. A dietitian can help give you a personalized recommendation. This will ensure you're able to get the right amount of fuel you require to maximize your results.

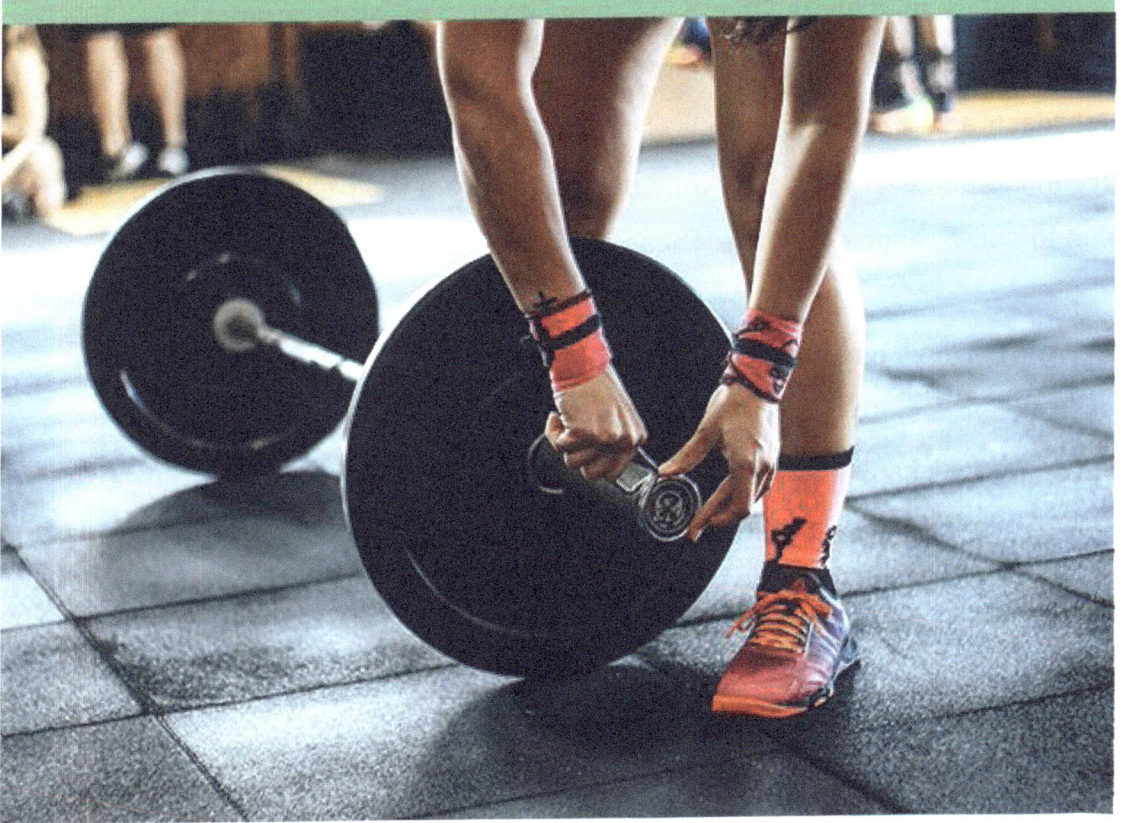

CHAPTER 7
TYPES OF CARB CYCLING

TYPES OF CARB CYCLING

Carb cycling represents an approach to dieting in which carb intake is alternated. There are no hard and fast rules about the basis on which you do this. Some people alternate daily, while others alternate on a monthly or weekly basis. Some people do long periods of high, moderate, and low carb diets. Others vary their approach on a day-to-day basis. This means that there is no single type of carb cycling to suit everyone. Everyone should program their carb intake. They can do this to suit a range of factors. These include:

- Your own body composition goals
- Your rest days and training days
- Your scheduled refeeds
- Whether you're attending a competition or special event
- The type of training you're undertaking and its intensity
- Your body fat level

Some carb cycling approaches involve two days of low carbs followed by a day of high carbs. This pattern repeats. Another approach is to have two days of high carb intake followed by two days of moderate carbs. There will then be three days of low carbs before returning to the beginning of the cycle. Usually, the protein intake will remain similar between all days.

Fat intake, meanwhile, will vary depending on the intake of carbohydrates. High carbohydrate days usually mean low-fat. Low carb days mean high fat. Another approach involves adjusting your carb intake week on week. For example, you may eat a low carb diet for 11 days in a row. You may then have high carbs for the following three days before returning to the beginning of the cycle. There is even a monthly adjustment approach. This involves eating low carbs for four weeks and then having a week of high carbs for the fifth week.

As you can see, there are many variations of carb cycling. That means some individual experimentation and trial and error will be required. Over time, you'll eventually find the right formula to suit you.

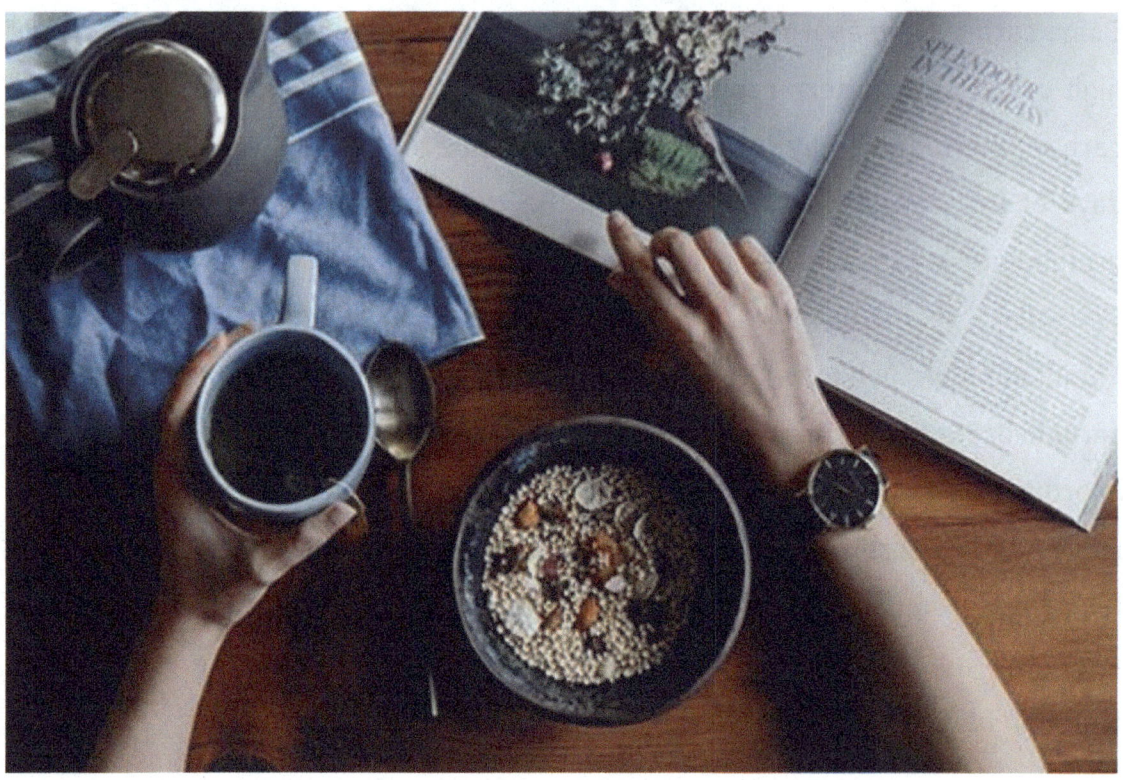

A quick overview of some of the most common carb cycling approaches is as follows:

- An infrequent, large refeed. This involves increasing carb intake every one to two weeks during a low carb intake phase.
- Moderate frequent refeeds. This involves increasing carb intake every three to four days in a low carb intake phase.
- Strategic carb cycling. This involves structuring menus with a moderate carb intake at specific, strategic intervals in a low carb intake phase. When you follow this approach, you'll steer away from a very high carb intake. It will, therefore, allow your metabolism to catch up to your dietary intake.
- Carb cycling to gain muscle. Anyone who wants to gain muscle mass will require a calorie surplus. However, when you overconsume calories in the

long-term, bodyfat gain is almost inevitable. Carb cycling allows muscle gain to be optimized over fat gain. Like strategic carb cycling, menus must be planned to match your weekly schedule. This will enable you to make a temporary surplus of calories to boost strength and lean mass gains.

CHAPTER 8

WHICH FOODS ARE GOOD ON A CARB CYCLING REGIME?

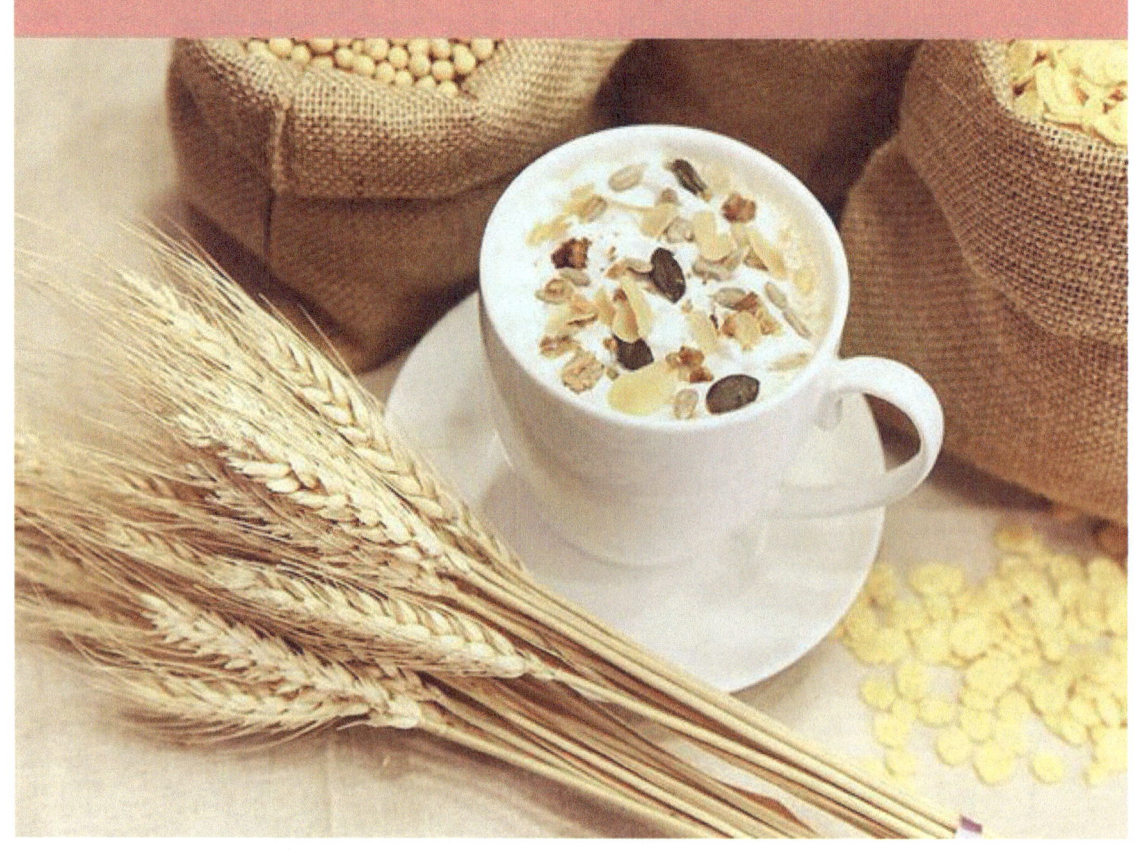

WHICH FOODS ARE GOOD ON A CARB CYCLING REGIME?

Before embarking on a carb cycling regime, you need to know more about what carbs are. You also need to know which ones are suitable to eat on this type of diet. Carbohydrates often have negative connotations. However, not all carbs are bad for you. Carbohydrates are essential in supplying energy. Here, we take a closer look at which ones you should be enjoying as part of your carb cycling lifestyle.

What Are Good Carbs?
Alongside fats and proteins, carbs are one of the three main macronutrients. Carbs are needed to supply energy to the brain and body. Whenever you eat carbs, they're broken-down during digestion into sugars. These sugars are then absorbed into the bloodstream. In response to the boost in blood sugar levels, the body releases insulin. It is needed to shuttle the sugar (called glucose at this stage) to the cells. This allows a quick energy boost to fuel activity.

Carbohydrates also get stored in the liver and muscles as glycogen. This is a stored type of glucose. However, excess glucose also gets stored as fat. Therefore, lots of people think that carbohydrates are bad for them. Not all carbohydrates are equal.

There are three primary types of carbohydrates: fiber, starch, and sugar. Sugar is by far the simplest type. Fiber and starch are both complex carbohydrates. This means they are more difficult to break down in the body. It takes longer and therefore you'll feel full for longer when you eat complex carbs. Processed or refined carbohydrates are less fibrous and starchy. They are more sugary and have less nutritional value.

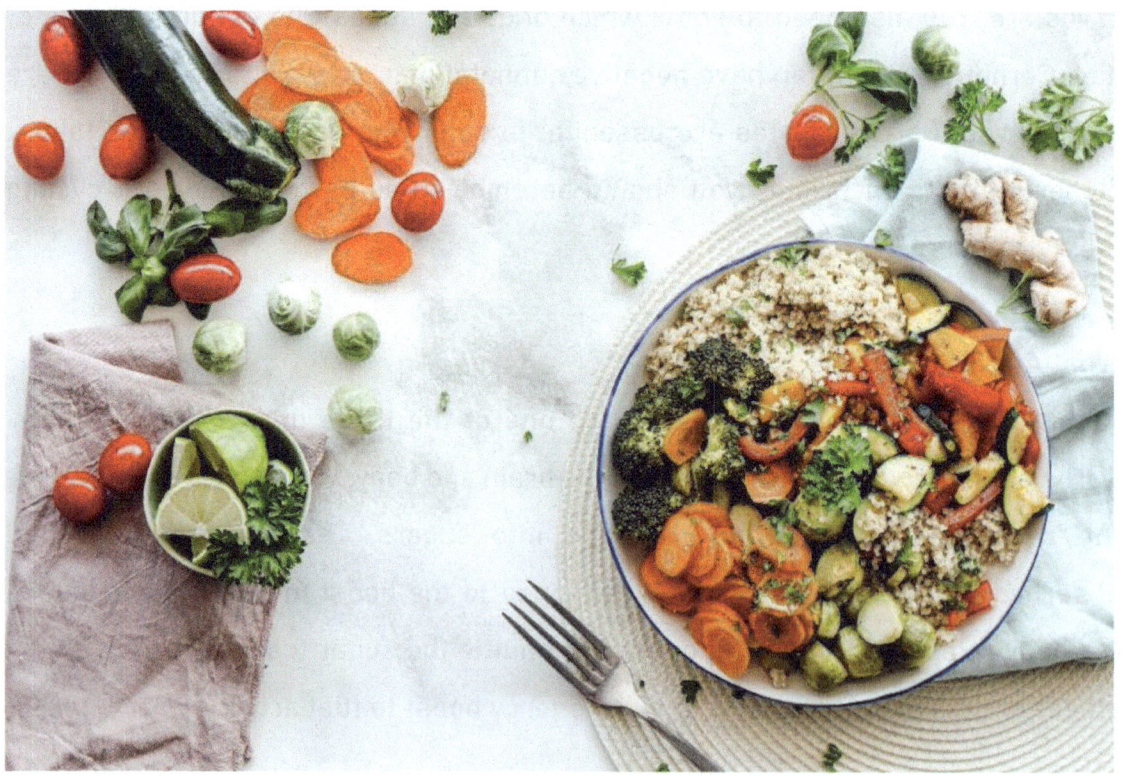

Processed carbs can be ditched from your diet when you're carb cycling.

However, whole foods that are rich in carbs should stay in your diet. Potatoes and starchy vegetables such as carrots and squash are complex carbohydrates which are good for you. Whole grains such as brown rice and quinoa and legumes such as lentils and beans are also good choices. Even foods containing natural sugars such as milk and fruit have a place in carb cycling diets.

These wholefoods have nutritional merits. They contain key minerals and vitamins. Therefore, although the word carbohydrates often produce images of sugary food that is unhealthy, this isn't always the case. Complex carbs have a vital role to play in ensuring you have a healthy lifestyle.

Of course, that doesn't mean that all carbohydrates can be included in a carb cycling diet. Some should always be avoided except as occasional treats. Yet there are lots of healthy sources of carbohydrate which have lots of beneficial minerals, vitamins, and fiber. They also taste great.

Therefore, when planning out a high carb day menu, you shouldn't see it as an excuse to binge on cookies. Instead, put your focus on healthy complex carb choices. Some recommended good carbohydrates include:

- Wholegrains – unmodified grains have many health benefits. They're very healthy and include quinoa, oats, and brown rice.
- Vegetables – all vegetables have different mineral and vitamin content. You should eat many different colors to obtain the right balance.
- Unprocessed fruit – like vegetables, all fruits are unique. Berries are especially healthy since they have a low glycemic load and a high antioxidant content.

- Legumes – these complex carbs are digested slowly. They are packed with minerals and fiber.
- Tubers – sweet potatoes and white potatoes are also complex carbs. They are slowly digested so you'll feel full for longer.

How do you identify which carbohydrates are good ones? They will be:
- High in fiber
- Unprocessed with no natural ingredients removed
- Slow to digest

Bad carbs, on the other hand will be:
- Found in very processed foods
- High in sugar
- Containing white flour
- Low in fiber content

What would be good examples of carbs to eat at each stage of your carb cycling plan?

On a no-carb day you should eat:
- Vegetables that are high in fiber like asparagus, leafy greens, mushrooms, and broccoli
- Lean protein
- Good fats

You should avoid eating:

- Starchy carbs. These include oats, rice, potatoes, and cereal. They also include starchy vegetables like squash, pumpkin, zucchini, and beans. Your total intake of carbs should be under 25 grams per day. All of these should come from fiber-filled vegetables.

On low carb days, you should eat:
- Fibrous vegetables
- Two to three servings of starch. All should be from clean sources like sweet potatoes, brown rice, fruit, starchy vegetables, and oats. They should be free from dairy, soy, and gluten. Starchy carbs should be eaten after your workout for the best results.

On high carbohydrate days you should eat:
- Up to 200 grams of carbs for a woman or 300 grams for a man. The total amount will vary to suit your activity level and size.
- Lots of lean protein.
- Plenty of healthy fats.

High carbohydrate days shouldn't be an excuse for binge eating. They are ways of systematically resetting your fat-burning and muscle-building hormones. Most of the fats should be from a clean source. However, if you're going to cheat, make sure to do it on one of these high carb days.

There are misconceptions that foods like pasta are banned from carb cycling diets. This isn't strictly true. If you put any food off limits, you'll just want to binge on it more. You can have foods like pasta.

However, if you're going to eat starchy foods that have little fiber and micronutrition you'll need to eat them strategically. You should only have them after you've worked out. This is because your insulin sensitivity will be highest at that time. Your body will, therefore, be able to use them at their best at this time. They're less likely to be converted into fat in the body and stored.

Good Fats and Proteins

On a high carb day, your focus should remain on complex carbs. You should avoid simple carbs. Complex carbohydrates help you stay full for longer. They all contain more nutrients and vitamins. On a no-carb day, you can't just cut out starch and sugar though. You need to replace those missing calories which you'd usually derive from carbs with something else. Good fats are a good substitute.

Of course, not all fats are good fats. Carb cycling is different from a keto diet. In the keto lifestyle, consuming all fats is encouraged. Even sources of saturated fat such as cheese and bacon can be eaten freely. On a carb cycling regime, these sources should be avoided. Good fats that are focused on omega-3 fatty acids can be eaten freely. You can find these in healthy sources such as avocados, chia seeds, fish, and olives.

Experts often recommend medium-chain triglycerides such as MCT oil on a carb cycling regime. These stimulate your neurological functions even on days when you're not eating carbs.

As well as good fats, you should make sure to eat plenty of lean protein. Protein contains no carbohydrates. Therefore, it can be eaten freely even on a no-carb day. Eggs, lean chicken, and fish are all good choices. They will help you feel full while boosting muscle growth.

CHAPTER 9
SAMPLE CARB CYCLING PROGRAMS

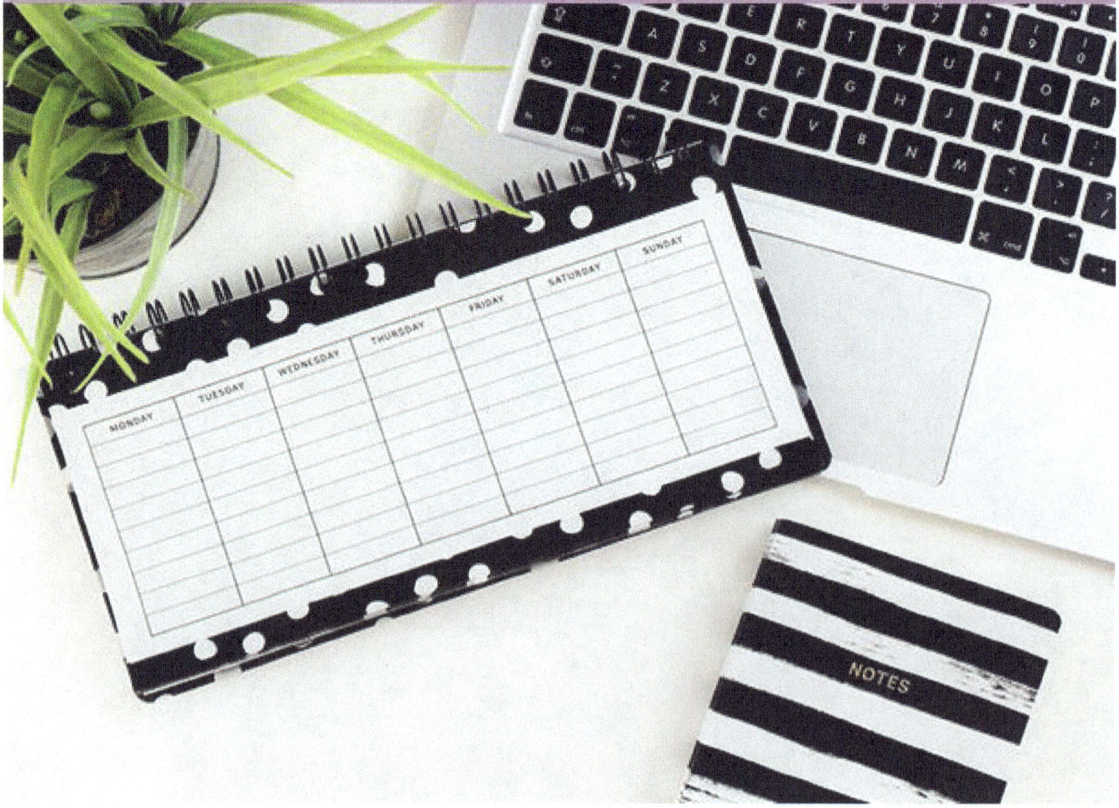

SAMPLE CARB CYCLING PROGRAMS

As we've already pointed out, there are many kinds of carb cycling program. This makes it hard to decide how you're going to go about getting started. If you're ready to put a carb cycling plan of your own in place, here are some sample regimes. They will help you to decide which work best for you.

Two of the most popular programs are:
- The High/Low Program
- The High/Medium/Low Program

Let's look at the High/Low Program first. This method involves having a high carbohydrate day then a low carb day. A high carbohydrate day involves eating more than 150 grams of carbs. A low carbohydrate day involves eating under 100 grams of carbs. The exact measurements and requirements will vary to suit each dieter. However, let's imagine we're planning a program for a 29-year-old female. Imagine she weighs 190 pounds and is 5 feet 8 inches tall. The total number of calories she needs to maintain weight is 190 x 15 i.e., 2850. She also weight trains three days a week. We're going to look at a few programs to suit her statistics to meet different goals.

Firstly, let's look at a suitable program for her if she wanted to lose fat. With this goal in mind, she would need three days of high carbohydrates. These would be at the level of calories required for maintenance. She would then follow this by four days of low carb eating. These four days would all be 600 calories below this maintenance figure. She would choose her three-weight training days as her high carbohydrate days. Her non-workout days would be her low carbohydrate days. Her program would, therefore, look something like this:

Training day intake – 2850 calories
Protein intake – 190 grams
Carbohydrate intake – 375 grams
Fat intake – 65 grams

Rest day intake – 2250 calories
Protein intake – 190 grams
Carbohydrate intake – 100 grams
Fat intake – 120 grams

Her total deficit of calories every week would be 600 x 4 i.e., 2400 calories. This would help her to lose just under 1 pound of fat every week. While this may not sound impressive, it's important to remember that rapid fat loss isn't the only goal. The more quickly fat is lost, the greater the chance of losing muscle too. This is the opposite of the aim of carb cycling. What about if the same individual wanted to try carb cycling to gain muscle?

In this case, her calorie intake needs to be adjusted slightly. She needs a surplus of calories in this instance. This will help her to recover after working out. It'll also promote more muscle tissue growth. Her goal is to have a surplus of 300 calories on her training days. On her low carb days, she will stay at her recommended maintenance intake. Her program would, therefore, look like this:

Training day intake – 3150 calories
Protein intake – 190 grams
Carbohydrate intake – 440 grams
Fat intake – 70 grams

Rest day intake – 2850 calories
Protein intake – 190 grams
Carbohydrate intake – 300 grams
Fat intake – 100 grams

You'll probably notice that the carb intake on a low carb day is surprisingly high. Earlier, we said the carb intake on a low carb day should be under 100 grams. Yet in this case, the individual has a high energy expenditure. Therefore, avoiding excess fat is important. Fat can be stored easily when there's a caloric surplus. Therefore, avoiding eating too much fat is important to prevent fat gain. Meanwhile, carbs are essential to refill muscle glycogen and promote recovery. This aids in training performance.

With this program, the individual is cycling carbs, however not so drastically as she would to lose weight. Some people find keeping carb intake to under 100g on their low carb days helps them to stay leaner. However, caloric intake must be kept at the same level overall, even on off days. This will ensure a net caloric surplus is maintained over the entire week. What about the high/medium/low method?

Well, this involves having a high carbohydrate day then a medium carbohydrate day. Finally, a low carbohydrate day will follow on. The cycle will then repeat. A high carbohydrate day involves eating over 150 grams of carbs. A medium carbohydrate day involves eating between 100 grams and 150 grams of carbs. A low carbohydrate day involves eating under 50 grams of carbs.

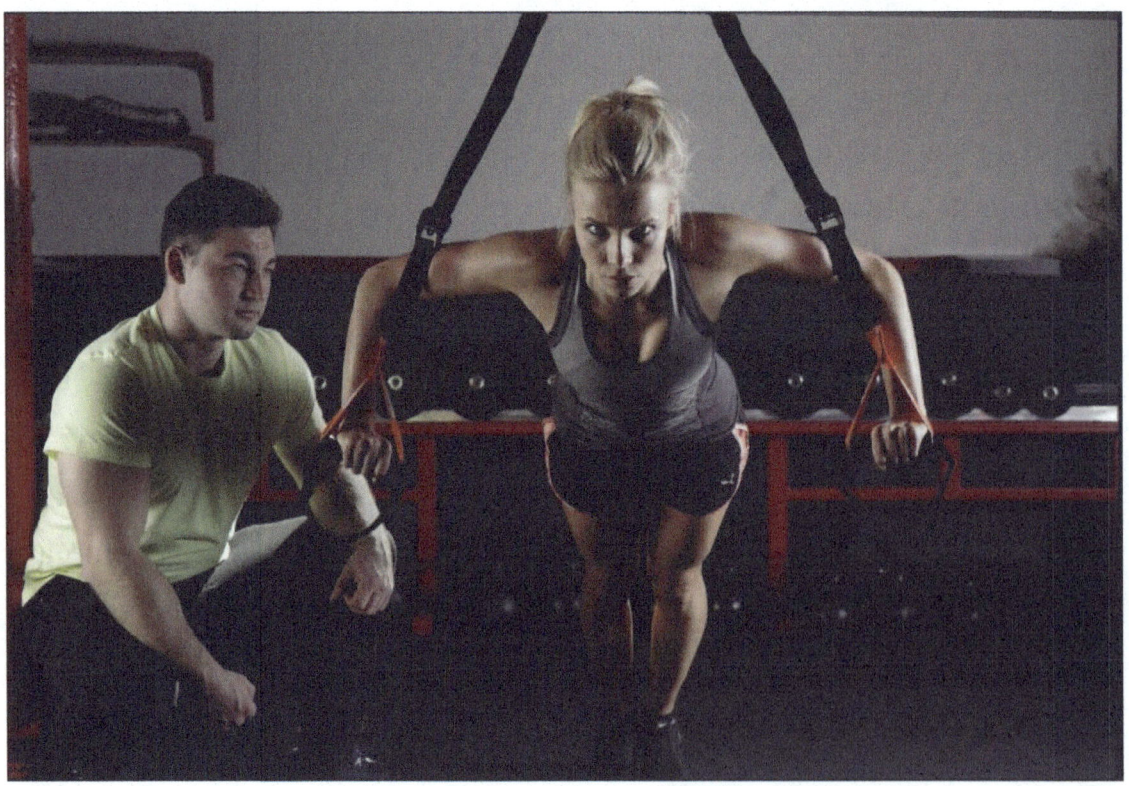

Now, let's imagine our dieter. She's a 31-year-old woman who is 5 feet 5 inches tall. She weighs 150 pounds and works out three days per week doing weight training. Her total calories for maintenance are 150 x 15 (2250).

If she wants to lose fat, this is a sample carb cycling plan for her. She should have two days of high carb intake. The calorie intake will be set at her maintenance level of 2250 calories. On her two medium carb days, her caloric intake will be 300 calories under this level. On her two low carb days, her caloric intake will be 600 calories under her maintenance level. Rather than aligning the high carbohydrate days with her training days, the intake is: staggered. Training should be carried out on medium and high carb days though, not low carb days. Her program will, therefore, look like this:

High carb day intake – 2250 calories
Protein intake – 150 grams
Carbohydrate intake – 245 grams
Fat intake – 75 grams

Medium carb day intake – 1950 calories
Protein intake – 150 grams
Carbohydrate intake – 150 grams
Fat intake – 80 grams

Low carb day intake – 1650 calories
Protein intake – 150 grams

Carbohydrate intake – 50 grams

Fat intake – 95 grams

Over the week, the plan could look like this:

Monday – training day – high carb

Tuesday – training day – medium carb

Wednesday – rest day – low carb

Thursday – training day – high carb

Friday – rest day – medium carb

Saturday – rest day – low carb

Sunday – rest day – low carb

If the same individual wanted to gain muscle through carb cycling, the plan would look different. A caloric surplus will be necessary so muscle tissue can grow and recover. Therefore, a 200-calorie surplus will be required on a training day. On rest days, she should eat the number of calories required for maintenance. Her program will, therefore, look like this:

High carb day intake – 2450 calories

Protein intake – 150 grams

Carbohydrate intake – 340 grams

Fat intake – 55 grams

Medium carb day intake – 2450 calories

Protein intake – 150 grams

Carbohydrate intake – 240 grams

Fat intake – 100 grams

Low carb day intake – 2250 calories
Protein intake – 150 grams
Carbohydrate intake – 150 grams
Fat intake – 115 grams

You may have noticed the medium carb day requirement is higher than suggested earlier. The same reasons apply in this case as applied in the above example. Eating excessive dietary fat in such circumstances can lead to the storage of fat. Therefore, avoiding eating too much fat helps to prevent fat gain. Carbs are vital in recovery and in refilling the muscle glycogen. This helps to boost training performance.

The individual in question here is still carb cycling. However, her plan isn't as drastic as it would be if she wanted to lose fat. If you use this method to gain muscle mass, you can adjust the carb and fat numbers to suit you. Some people find if they keep their carbohydrates to under 100g on rest days, they stay leaner. This may work for you, but you'll still need your caloric intake to remain at the maintenance level even on rest days. This will ensure you're in a caloric surplus overall during the week.

The key nutrient for maintaining and gaining muscle is protein. Nevertheless, it doesn't have to be exceptionally high, whether you want to gain muscle or reduce fat. 1g of protein for each pound of your bodyweight is ideal. Fat and carb totals are important too. However, they can be tailored to your energy expenditure and preferences.

How about if you want to maintain your bodyweight? You can still achieve this goal with carb cycling. You simply need to choose one of the above methods. You then adjust your rest day and training day intakes, so they balance out over the week. One way of doing this is to consume 200 calories more than your recommended maintenance level on a training day. On a rest day, you should have 200 calories under this figure. So, if your maintenance intake is 2500 calories, you'd have 2700 on training days and 2300 on a rest day.

CHAPTER 10

HOW DO I GET STARTED WITH CARB CYCLING?

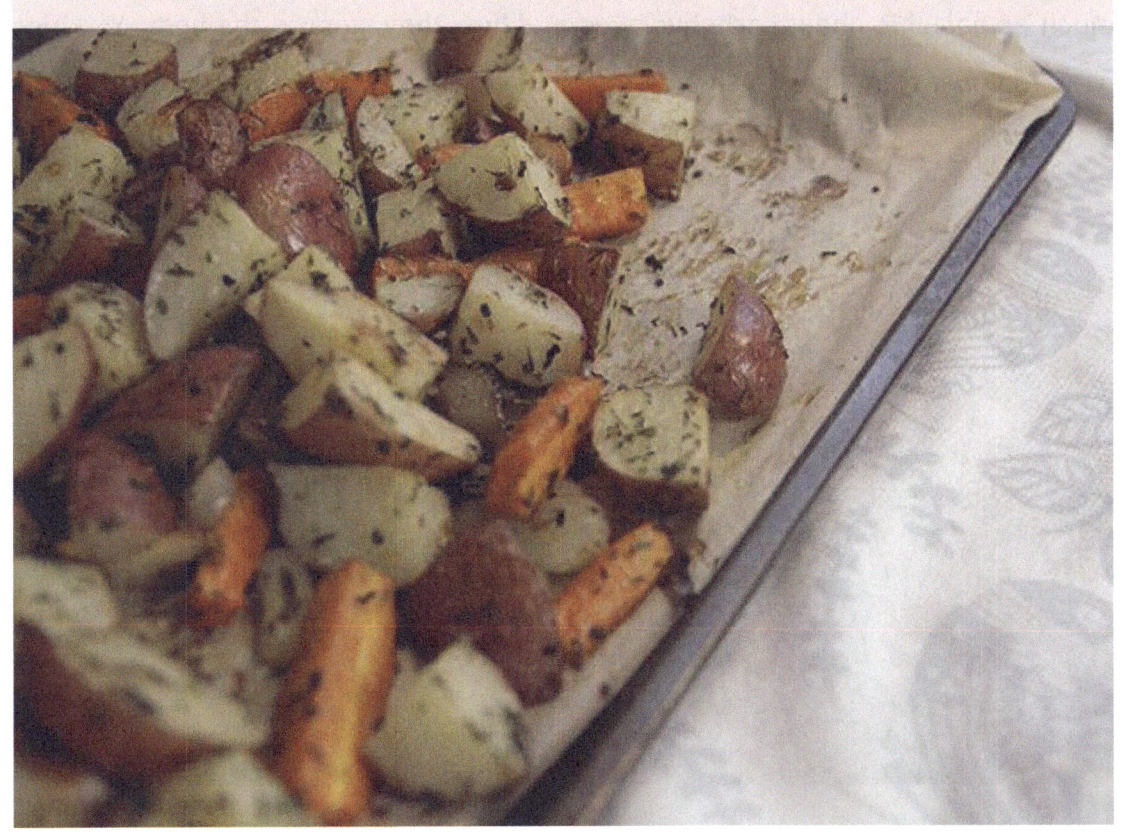

HOW DO I GET STARTED WITH CARB CYCLING?

Although the idea of carb cycling is appealing, it's difficult to know how to get started. This way of eating can be quite complex. Therefore, you need to know as much as possible about carbohydrates and how they work in the body. You also need to understand how to choose the right carb cycling plan for you.

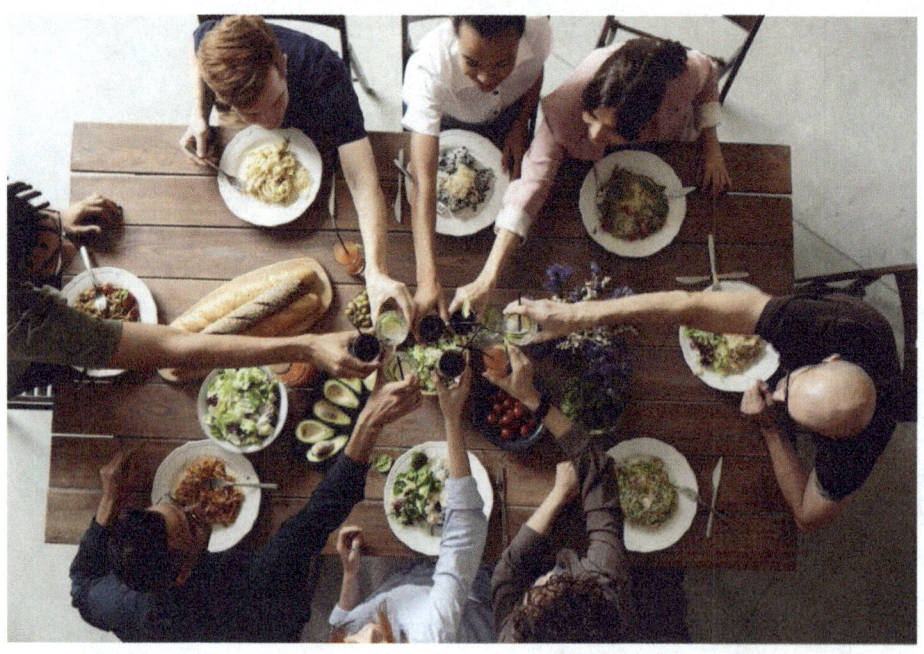

The information we've provided in the earlier chapters will help you to determine the right program for you. However, you could probably benefit from a few expert tips to get you off to the right start. Here is some good advice to point you in the right direction. First, we'll look at how to avoid the major pitfalls of carb cycling. Here are some of the most common:

- Focusing solely on carbs while ignoring other macros. Some people are confused by the name "carb cycling". It's a misnomer. Carb cycling isn't only about carbohydrates. It's about balancing your calorie intake over the week. If carb intakes are lowered on a rest day, more protein and fat need to be eaten to compensate. It's only by doing this that fat loss can be maintained in the long term.

You need to know the number of calories you need to consume to maintain weight first. This enables you to plan how much you need to adjust your intake to suit each rest or training day. On a rest day, take 10 percent to 20 percent off your calorie intake from carbohydrates but don't increase your protein or fat intake. There are four calories in each gram of carbohydrate. Therefore, if you eat two thousand calories each day, cut your intake of carbs by 50 grams on rest days.

- Your calorie intake is varying too much. The 10 percent to 20 percent rule specifically applies to carbs. However, you shouldn't ever have over 33 percent difference in the total amount of calories consumed over the week. Too much variance hurts recovery. It also makes it more difficult to adhere to the carb cycling regime. You can remedy this by eating a minimum of 68 percent of your usual energy intake on low carb days.

- You're using your high carb days as a cheat day. High output days aren't an excuse to eat anything you like. If you do this regularly, unhealthy eating habits start to set in. You can fix this by focusing mainly on foods that are dense in nutrients. Eat more whole foods such as oats and potatoes on your high carb days. Eat more nuts and eggs on your low carb days. You'll feel full but won't ruin your overall regime. Now you know what to avoid, here are some tips for every carb cycling program.
- Base your chosen dietary approach on your activity level and basal calorie needs.
- Choose your refeed days well in advance.
- Always adhere to your regime until your refeeding day.
- Keep all your decisions based on the outcome. Different strategies for refeeding work best for different body types. You should take body composition tests to check you're on the best track for you.
- Exercise on your refeeding days. This will ensure the best body composition results.
On refeed days eat more carbs in the morning and at times when you're doing a lot of physical activity.
- On low carbohydrate days, eat more leafy greens. They are virtually free of calories but add more bulk to your plate. You'll find a full-looking plate more satisfying.
- Eat wholefood fats on low carb days. Cold water fish, nuts, grass-fed butter, eggs, avocado, and coconut oil are all good choices.
- Measure your carbs and fats. This will help you to track how many calories you consume. On a normal day, measure your carbs too. A lot of the time, we underestimate how much protein we're eating and overestimate the

amount of fat and carbs.

- Don't reduce carbs without eating more fat. Your body requires either fats or carbs for energy. That means you'll need to fuel up for the day in one way or the other.
- Avoid skipping meals. You might be tempted to avoid eating to lose more weight on normal or low carb days. This is a bad idea. It could result in your body breaking down more muscle.
- Avoid winging it. Deciding to try carb cycling is very different to the reality of doing it. You'll need to be dedicated and keep detailed records of your intake at each meal. You'll need to do this every day for weeks on end. There's no way to look at an ingredient and know its calorie and macronutrient contents. Therefore, you'll need to measure and record accordingly. Apps such as MyPlate and My Fitness Pal are good for this.
- Always choose foods that support your overall well-being, even on high carb days. Huge mounds of pasta and white bread, gallons of sugary drinks and tons of cake won't help your health. Opt for complex carbs that are rich in fiber instead. Quinoa, wholegrain bread, and oatmeal are all filling and satisfying. They're also good for your health.
- Indulge occasionally. Just because you should be eating healthily most of the time doesn't mean you can never indulge. If you forbid yourself from eating desserts or bagels, you'll just end up craving them. As a result, you'll end up cheating more and ruining your diet. It could also lead to a damaging relationship with eating and food over time. If you choose complex carbs on most high carb days, you can have the odd cookie or candy bar.
- Talk to an expert. Nutrition can be a complex subject, nuanced for everyone. Working closely with a professional could, therefore, be a good

idea. A nutritionist will be able to draw up a personalized diet plan which is based on your needs. It will be tailored to suit your specifications, your goals and your activity level. This will ensure you get all the right nutrients but still achieve your chosen outcomes.

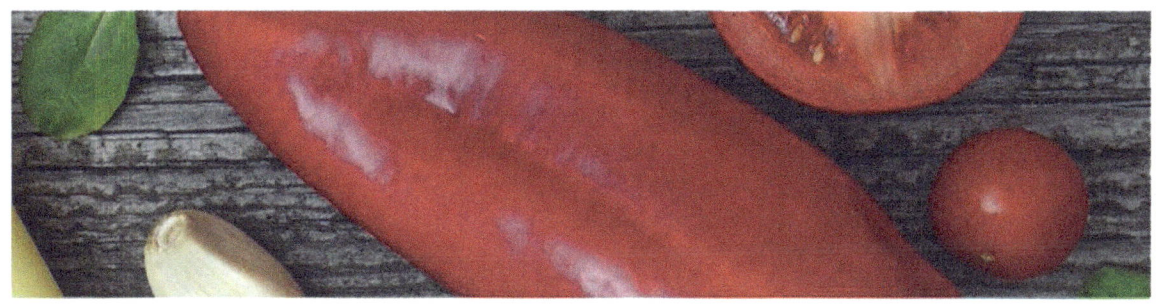

CARB CYCLING MADE EASY

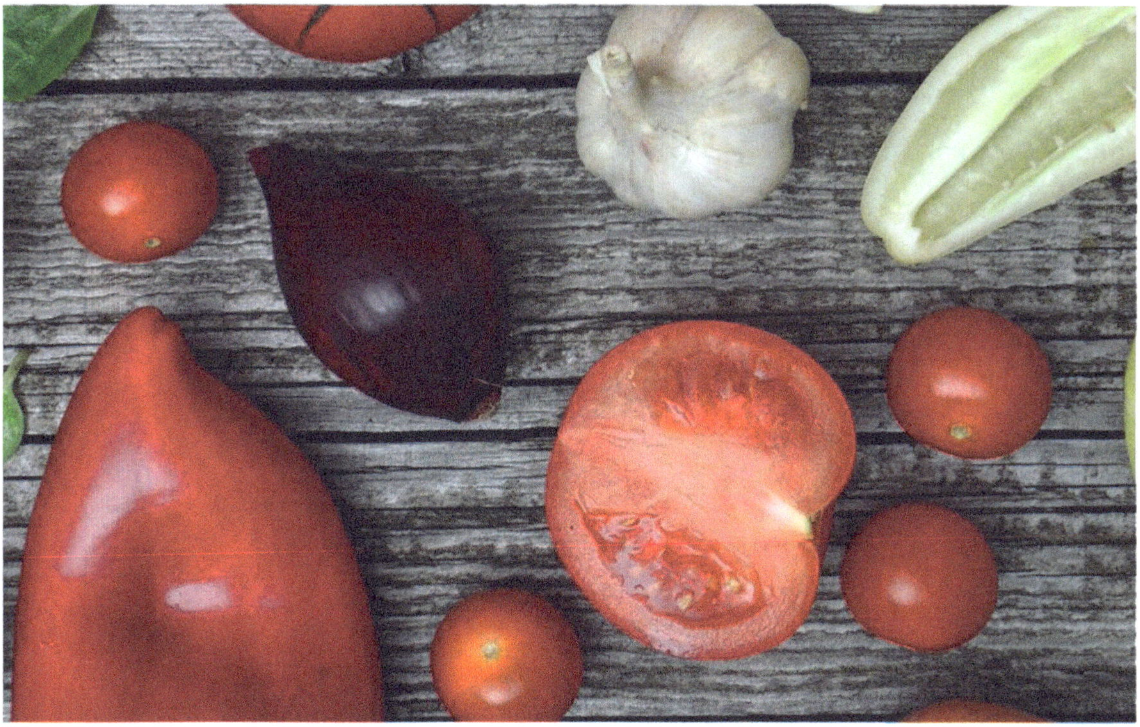

CARB CYCLING MADE EASY – MEAL PLANS

Putting all this information into a concrete meal plan can be daunting for beginners. These additional sample meal plans for a typical carb cycling week should help. Use them along with the others previously mentioned, as a basic blueprint for designing your meals but remember, it's not carved in stone. You can add or discard meals according to your chosen 7-day plan.

PLAN 1

Monday (low carb day)

Breakfast
3 whole eggs, scrambled, poached boiled or fried.
1/2 cup of high-carb fruit like blueberries, pineapple or peaches
1/cup oatmeal sweetened with honey

Snack
I apple or 1/2 cup unsalted nuts

Lunch

Turkey sandwich with lettuce and tomato on wholewheat bread.

Herbal tea

Snack

1/2 cup ricotta cheese or 2 medium apricots

Dinner

Spinach Frittata

Grilled beef strips with green bell peppers

Green salad

Tuesday (High carb day)

Breakfast

Two slices whole wheat bread with Swiss cheese

1 cup low-fat yogurt with fresh blueberries

Snack

1 banana

Lunch

Grilled salmon with brown rice

Grated carrot and cucumber salad

Snack

1 slice whole wheat bread with almond butter

Dinner

Whole wheat pasta with fresh tomatoes

Black beans with garlic oil

Fresh green salad

Wednesday (low carb day)

Breakfast

3 scrambled eggs with avocado

Snack

2 apricots or 2 plums

Lunch

Caesar salad with grilled chicken strips

Herbal tea

Snack

Low-fat yogurt or 1/2 cup of nuts

Dinner

Flank steak with green beans and onions

Green salad with feta cheese

Thursday (High carb day)

Breakfast
2 poached eggs
2 slices whole-wheat toast
1/2 cup fruit

Snack
1/2 cup fruit or nuts or 1 banana

Lunch
1 cup brown rice with chickpeas
Sweet potatoes
Green salad

Snack
Low-fat yogurt with honey or 1 banana

Dinner
Baked potato
Grilled chicken breast
Avocado and tomato salad

Friday (low carb day)

Breakfast

1/2 cup oatmeal

1/2 cup fruit

1/2 cup ricotta, feta, or goat cheese

Snack

1/2 cup fruit or nuts or 1 low-fat yogurt

Lunch

Avocado and chicken salad

Sliced tomatoes on lettuce

Herbal tea

Snack

1 orange or 1 apple or 2 plums

Dinner

Grilled salmon with vegetables

Naked beans

Green salad

Saturday (high carb day)

Breakfast

2 scrambled eggs on whole-wheat toast

1 low-fat yogurt sweetened with honey

Lunch

Sweet potatoes

Lentil soup

Snack

1/2 cup nuts or fruit

Dinner

Tuna Casserole Whole wheat noodles

Spinach salad

Sunday (low carb + cheat day)

Breakfast

Lean sausages with fried eggs

1/2 cup fruit

Snack

Almond butter or 1/2 cup nuts

Lunch

Tuna salad

1 piece of fresh fruit

Snack

2 plums, two apricots or 1 apple

Dinner:

Whatever you want! In moderation, please. For example, have two slices of pizza instead of three or four. Indulge in a moderate portion of ice cream or cake. If you've been craving French fries all week, eat a small portion of them, not a whole platter. You get the idea.

PLAN 2

If you prefer more than three meals a day, here is a sample plan to guide you.

TYPICAL LOW CARB DAY

Meal 1

3 scrambled or boiled eggs

3 strips of lean bacon

Sautéed peppers

Meal 2

4 oz. grilled turkey or chicken breast

1 cup carrots

Lettuce and tomato salad

Meal 3

4 Oz grilled salmon or tuna

1 cup broccoli

1 banana

Meal 4

4 oz. chicken

1 cup spinach

1 low-fat yogurt with honey

Meal 5

4 oz. tuna

1 cup chickpeas

1 sliced tomato or cucumber

Meal 6

4 oz. lean steak

1 cup green beans

1/2 cup fruit

TYPICAL HIGH CARB DAY

Meal 1

2 eggs

3 strips of bacon or 3 small sausages

2 slices whole-wheat toast

Meal 2

4 oz. chicken

Green salad

1/2 cup oatmeal sweetened with honey

Meal 3

4 oz. salmon

1/2 cup brown rice

1/2 cup carrots and peas

Meal 4

4 oz. chicken

2 cups spinach

1 cup arb-rich fruit like peaches, plums or apricots

Meal 5

1 cup of corn

1 sliced cucumber

1/2 cup of wild rice or quinoa

Meal 6

4 oz. grilled beefsteak

1 yam

1 cup green beans

Green salad

PLAN 3

Here is a third meal plan sample that just includes several suggestions for each day, letting you calculate the portions as you will learn below.

Recommended Food Portions

In addition to calorie and gram intake, the recommended quantities for carbs, some meal plans include portions in half-cups or cups (if you are using meal plans you found online for example). This is perfectly fine. There is no need for complicated conversions. Notice that on low carb days, your fat and protein intake will be higher. Make sure you are eating healthy fats and proteins. Invest in a small food scale easily measure gram and oz. portions. To follow is the recommended daily intake of carbs, proteins, and fats.

High Carb Days

Carbs	2 – 2.5 gm.
Proteins	1 gm.
Fats	0 -0.15 gm.-

Low Carb Days

Carbs	0.5 gm.
Proteins	1.5 gm
Fats	0.35

Low carb day

Breakfast

Egg muffins

Sour cream with chives

1 banana

OR…

Whole wheat pancakes with cream cheese

3 sausages

Blueberries or diced pineapple

OR…

3 scrambled eggs with green peppers and tomatoes

Vanilla yogurt with sliced banana

Lunch

Tacos with lean ground beef

Green salad

1-piece whole fruit

OR…

Bell peppers stuffed with lean ground beef

Sliced cucumber and spinach topped with grated parmesan cheese

1 apple

OR…

Chicken salad on lettuce

Baked butternut squash with herbs

Fruit salad

Dinner

Whole wheat pasta with grilled chicken strips and parmesan cheese

Green beans with carrots

Oatmeal sweetened with honey

OR…

Beef stroganoff with mushrooms

Brown rice

Shredded lettuce and tomato salad

Jelly cup

OR…

Chicken fajita wraps

Zucchini boats stuffed with mozzarella

Green salad

1-piece whole fruit

Snacks

Rice cake with almond butter

Protein shake

Hummus dip and celery sticks

Strawberry and banana smoothie

Cottage cheese with honey

Cream cheese with herbs and carrot sticks

HIGH CARB DAYS

Breakfast

Scrambled eggs with bacon and chives

Oatmeal with blueberries and honey

1-piece whole fruit

OR…

Boiled eggs

2 slices whole-wheat bread with cream cheese

1 banana

OR…

Fried eggs with sausage

2 slices whole what toast

1 yam

Lunch

Grilled turkey sandwich

Chickpea salad

Yogurt with honey

OR…

Grilled salmon

Sweet potato and spinach salad

1-piece whole fruit

OR…

Fish or tuna with whole wheat noodles

Potato salad

1-piece whole fruit

Dinner:

Baked chicken

Mexican brown rice

Peas with carrots

1-piece whole fruit

OR…

Pan steak with potatoes

Broccoli with sweet corn

Jelly cup

OR…

Pasta with chicken and mushroom

Cherry tomato and spinach salad

Quinoa sweetened with honey

As you can see, there is huge room to get creative and once up with mouthwatering, meals. Once you get the hang of it, you will be able to come up with delicious treats for the whole family to enjoy along with you (although family members not on the plan or kids should not restrict themselves to portions or calories. You can also tweak your favorite recipes to make them carb cycling-friendly by replacing processed carbs with healthy ones, and saturated fats with good fats.

Conclusion

As you can see, there are many advantages associated with carb cycling. Nevertheless, it is not a diet regime for everyone. You need to be dedicated and committed to your goals to see it through. Carb cycling is ideal for anyone who knows what they want to achieve from their diet. There are a few things you need to do before you get started though. You will need to know your maintenance caloric intake. This will be based on your activity level, gender, age, and height. When you have this figure, you need to pair it with your desired outcome.

It is then relatively simple to work out the right plan for you. Whether you want to lose weight, gain muscle or both, carb cycling could be ideal for you. If you've recently lost weight and want to maintain it, it is also useful for you. You simply need to select the right carb cycling plan to suit your schedule. Align your high and low carb days with your activity level and physique goals. You can then use the information provided in this guide to choose suitable foods for you.

Remember that you need to choose the right dietary intake every day when you are carb cycling. You cannot just indulge in sugary and starchy foods when you feel like it. While you can have an occasional treat, you mainly need to focus on complex carbs. Making sure to keep your protein and fat intake level constant every day of the week is also important.

With the right approach, you could find that carb cycling is the weight loss solution you have been looking for.

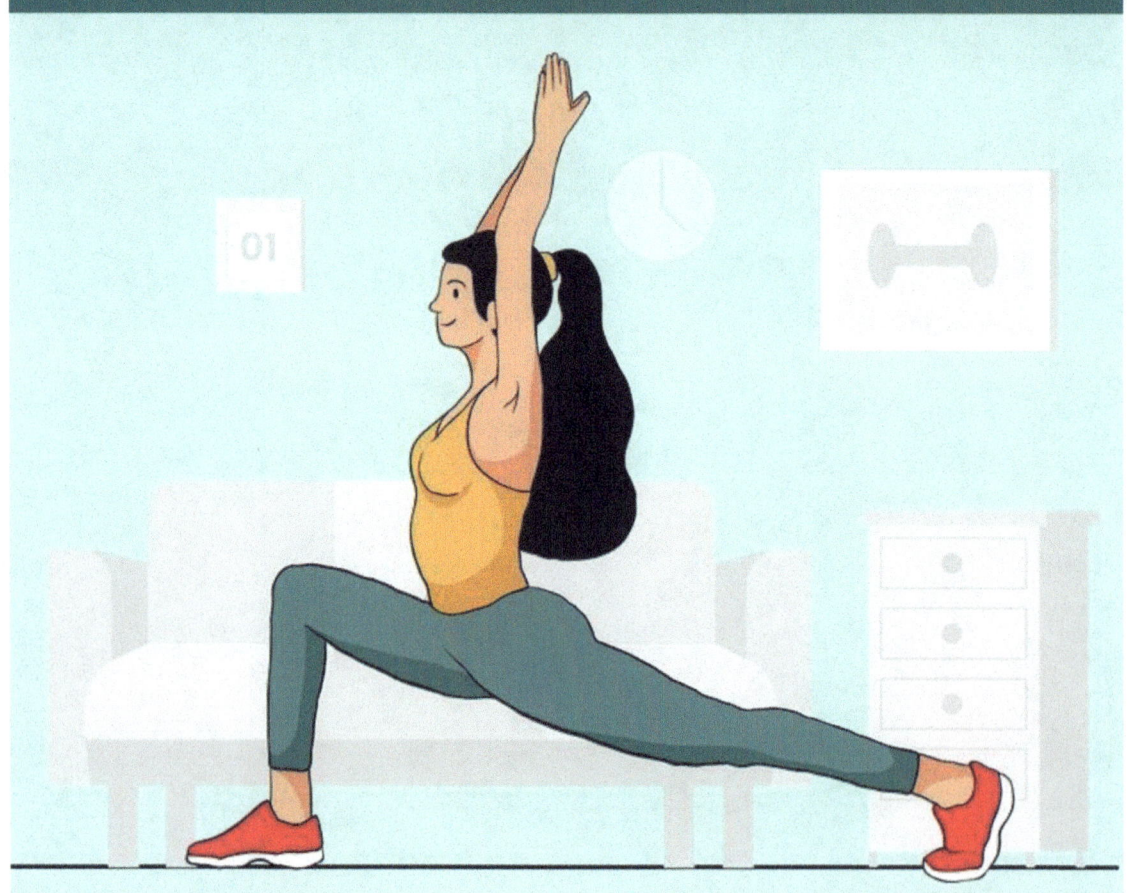

HOME BASED TRAINING:

HOW TO START WORKING OUT AT HOME FOR BEGINNERS

When was the last time you did squats? High school PE class? Or maybe you tried strength training as part of a home workout plan a few months ago but lost your motivation? No matter how far you are now from your desired fitness level...

Remember this:

It just takes one second to decide you're worth it, 10 minutes for your first workout, and two weeks to feel a difference.

Everything you need to know about how to start exercising and maintaining your workout routine is summed up in this helpful guide:

What you need to know before you begin (benefits of exercise)

Almost everyone knows exercise improves your health. However, a lot of people aren't aware of all the benefits of exercise.

Top benefits you can look forward to when you start working out:
- Reduced risk of chronic disease
- Better mood & mental health
- Balanced energy levels throughout the day & better sleep
- Slowing of the aging process

- A boost to brain health
- Positive effect on the microbiome
- A boost to sex life

How much exercise is recommended weekly for health benefits?

The general exercise recommendation is:
- Cardio (minimum amount of activity): At least 150 minutes of moderate cardio throughout the week. It can be replaced with at least 75 minutes of intense cardio throughout the week or a combination of both.
- Strength training (highly recommended): Exercises involving major muscle groups on two or more days a week.
- For extra health benefits: Minimum cardio should be increased by an additional 300 minutes per week (moderate) or 150 minutes of (intense) cardio per week (or a combination of both).

While it may sound like a lot, the good thing is that you can adjust this to your schedule and even do them as part of a home workout plan. As long as the cardio activities are performed for at least 10 minutes, you can divide your active minutes into as many workout sessions you like per week. Whether you do strength or cardio first depends on your goal.

Types of Exercise
What are some common types of exercise?
Cardio: Anything that raises your heart rate and makes you breathe faster can be considered cardio. However, it usually refers to activities aimed at improving your endurance and stamina such as:
- Moderate cardio: Brisk walking, dancing, jogging, cycling, swimming

- Intense cardio: Running, fast cycling, brisk walk up a hill, swimming laps
- Strength training: Any type of activity that uses resistance to build muscular strength. Using your own bodyweight as resistance has many benefits!
- Flexibility & mobility training: Exercises focused on maintaining and improving passive range of motion (flexibility) and active range of motion during movement (mobility).
- HIIT: HIIT or high-intensity interval training consists of intense bursts of exercise (strength or cardio) followed by rest intervals, aimed at keeping your heart rate elevated. Find out more about the difference between low-intensity, steady-state cardio, and HIIT cardio.

What is the best type of exercise to lose weight?

Any type of exercise that requires high effort (for you) will have a similar effect – especially for beginners. So, the truth is, it does not really matter! Find activities that you enjoy and can imagine doing for more than just a month or two. In the end, weight loss is about calorie deficit. So, make sure to adjust your nutrition for best results.

Tips on how to start exercising

First step: reach the fitness level where you don't feel like you "hate exercise" anymore. Here's how to do it…

Choose your inspiration and set a goal

How many times have you decided to start a home workout plan to lose 5 kg and then failed? Take a different approach and decide what you want to get good at first. Think of what you want to be able to do – whether it's getting into better shape, so you are more energized and productive at work or keeping up with your kids as you get older. Find your inspiration and then set yourself long-term and short-term goals.

Start small and track your progress
Starting small means focusing on short term goals first.

Focus on one week at a time. Get in your workout for the day. Then complete the next workout. Make it a challenge to find that 15-45 minutes in your day, as often as possible, to just get more active.

Once the first week is finished, look back and take it a step further – aim for one more workout or just five additional minutes of cardio in the next week.

Establishing a workout routine and sticking to it is more important than the duration & type of workouts you are doing. On days when you really have no time, even short 7-10-minute workouts can provide health benefits, especially for beginners.

It takes time to see results. Try to keep track of your progress from the start, so you can see how you improve day by day and stay motivated. Running apps can help you keep an eye on your progress and support you on your fitness journey – from the first workout to your first completed training plan. Be proud of every active minute that you add to your schedule!

Expect setbacks and have a Plan B
Skipping a workout or getting a cold shouldn't throw you off your game. Everyone experiences setbacks. Often even after the first 2-3 weeks.

"The goal is not to be perfect, but to get better with time. The important thing is that you don't give up. Just like you don't quit school because of a bad grade or don't quit your job when you face a challenge"

Here are some options for what to do when you experience a setback:
- Planned a workout but suddenly feel like you have no energy at all? If you already feel exhausted in the morning, take a break from exercising and really focus on what you eat during this rest day to improve your nutrition. If you start feeling too tired later in the afternoon, do a quick, easy workout to relax and get some movement in your day.
- Feeling stressed or lost motivation for your workout plan? It's normal to get overwhelmed. Skip a day and focus on getting a quality night of sleep.
- Skipped a couple of days and now you feel bad? Think about what caused this – was it a cheat meal, a tough day, or just a packed schedule? Learn something from it because it will happen again. Prepare yourself to continue where you left off. Every setback can bring new insights and motivation if you are ready to look deeper

Extra tips for beginners

Check your health: It's always good to get advice from your doctor or physical therapist before making big changes to your lifestyle, such as starting a new workout routine – especially if you are over 45, suffer from any chronic illness, or had injuries in the past. Don't exhaust yourself right away: No pain, no gain? Should you really be pushing yourself as a beginner? Yes, but only for the sake of consistency. Push yourself to be more active, but don't do an exercise when you are in pain. The real battle is in your head, and it's about getting through the first months. Once you make it a habit and learn how to perform all the exercises, it's time to push yourself even harder in your workouts.
Think about your form: Avoid injury and get better results by learning from common exercise mistakes. When you start working out, it might feel overwhelming to consider so many tips on form. Focus on getting better in one exercise every couple of days, not

all at once. And if you don't feel ready to perform a certain exercise – don't force it. There are always other options and ways to replace exercises with easier variations. Do what you can with good form and be patient: strength and endurance come with consistency!

A rep range for every goal

Remember before you exercise to determine your goal which in will influence how you train and its frequency.

TO LOSE WEIGHT

Sets: 4
Reps: 8
Intensity: 1–2 reps shy of failure
Equipment: Free weights, bodyweight or machines

When people want to lose weight, they automatically assume they should do light weights for tons of reps. Unfortunately, it doesn't work that way. To lose weight, you're likely be in a caloric deficit (i.e. eating fewer calories than you're burning), which means you won't have a ton of energy reserved to do high reps. Instead, stick to moderate weight and moderate reps. Heavier weights also give your body a reason to hang on to hard-earned muscle as you lose weight.

TO GET REALLY STRONG

Sets: 5
Reps: 3–5
Intensity: 2–3 reps shy of failure
Equipment: Mostly free weights (but some machines are OK, too)

There's no sugar coating it; getting strong takes a lot of work. And by work, we mean lifting progressively heavier weights over time. Skip the light dumbbells and sets of 20. Instead, opt for big free-weight exercises that use lots of muscles (like squats, deadlifts and rows) and stick with lower rep ranges. Because you'll be using more complicated exercises, stop each set 2-3 reps shy of failure to ensure your technique is on point.

TO BUILD MUSCLE

Sets: 3
Reps: 8, 10, 12
Intensity: 1 rep shy of failure
Equipment: Free weights or machines

While heavy weights are best for getting stronger, building muscle requires a little more finesse. As hokey as it sounds, the "mind-muscle" connection is very real. Use lighter weights and focus on feeling the target muscle squeezing and burning. Use the same weight for each set, but gradually increase the reps each set until you're just shy of failure. This laser-like focus leads to rapid gains in muscle tone and size.

TO RUN FASTER AND JUMP HIGHER

Sets: 8-10
Reps: 3
Intensity: Light to moderate (but move the weight as fast as possible)
Equipment: Free weights

Running faster and jumping higher requires more efficient recruitment of fast-twitch muscle fibers. While it's usually best to lift weights in a slow, controlled manner, lifting weights explosively targets your fast-twitch fibers to make you faster and more athletic. Use lower-body free-weight exercises like squats or kettlebell swings and keep the reps low so you can put everything you have into every set. And finally, don't go too heavy; if the weight isn't moving quickly, lighten the load.

TO BUILD ENDURANCE

Sets: 1

Reps: 12 or more
Intensity: Failure (keep going until you can't do any more reps)
Equipment: Machines

Sometimes one set is all it takes. If endurance is the name of the game, it's likely you're using strength training as cross-training for a sport like running, cycling or swimming. Being brutally strong isn't all that important, so pick a weight, do as many reps as you can (ideally 12 or more) and move on to the next exercise. Machines work best for training to failure since you're less likely to use poor technique compared to free-weight exercises.

Simple body weight exercises to be done at home

Look at the pictures and follow in the appropriate rep ranges according to goal

Stretching

FROG STRETCH

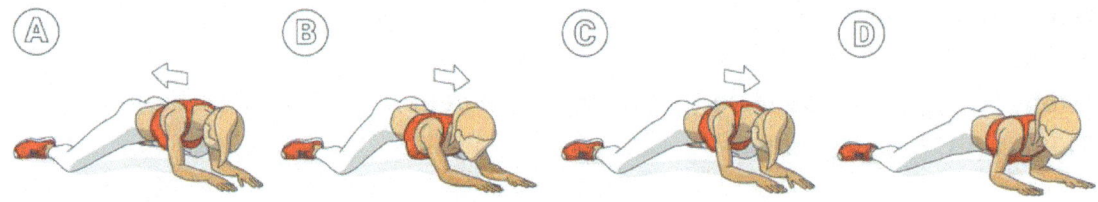

QUADRICEPS STRETCH
STANDING VARIATION

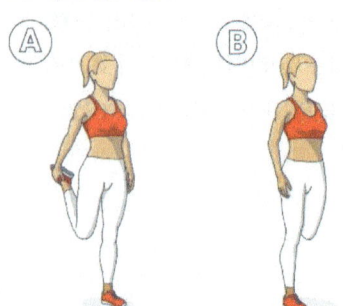

FORWARD BEND
easy variation
WITH YOGA STRAP

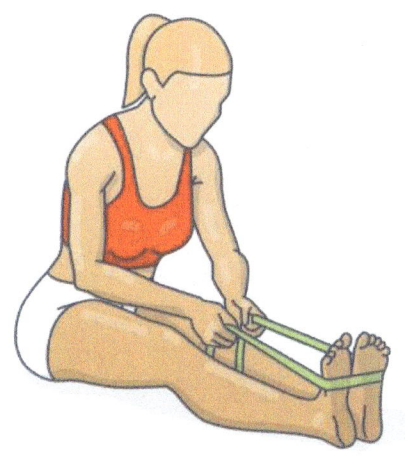

FORWARD HEAD TO KNEE
easy variation
WITH YOGA STRAP

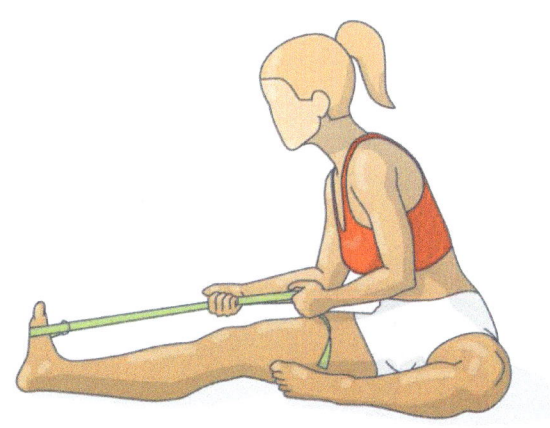

LEG STRETCHING
LEFT & RIGHT SIDE

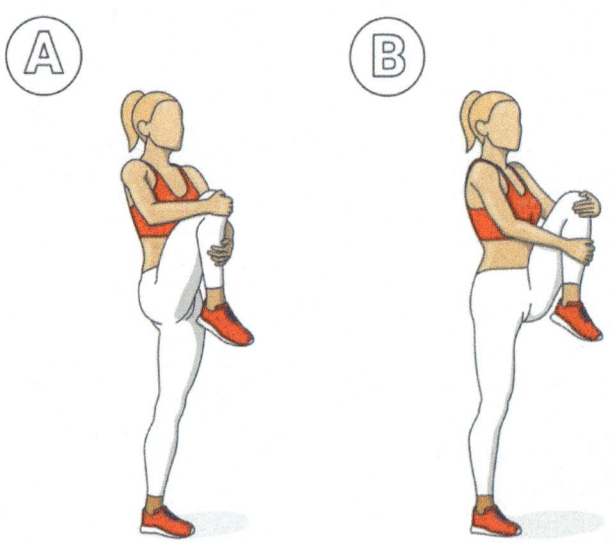

REVOLVED HEAD TO KNEE
easy variation
WITH YOGA STRAP

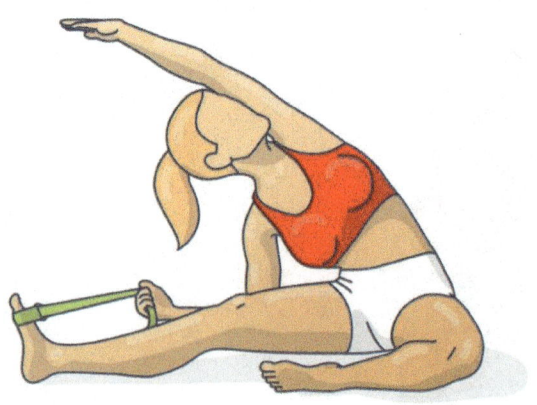

Full body range motion (aim for 30 – 60 seconds)

JUMPING JACKS

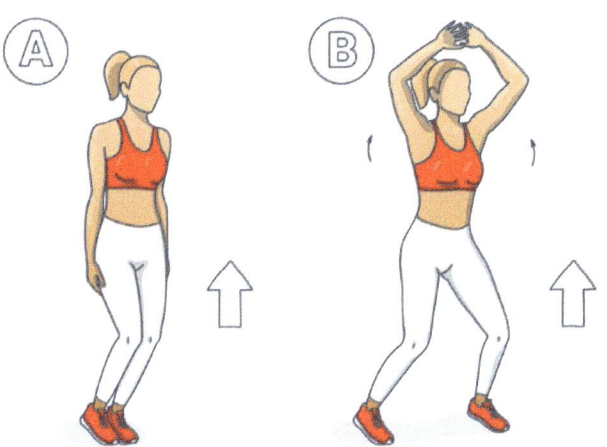

MOUNTAIN CLIMBERS
STANDING VARIATION

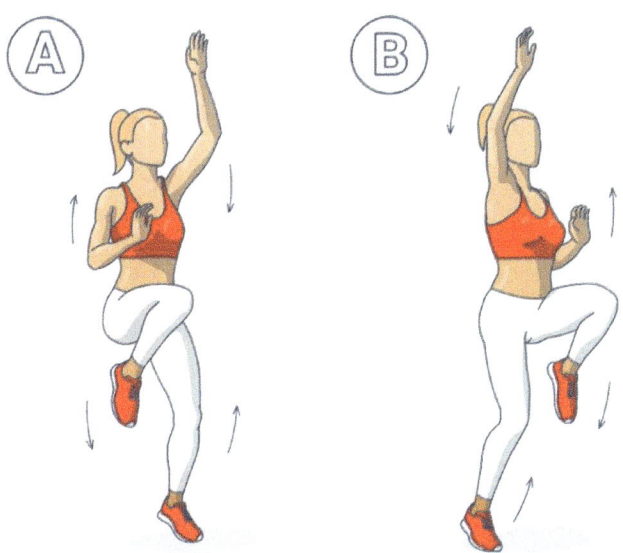

BURPEE
OR SQUAT THRUST

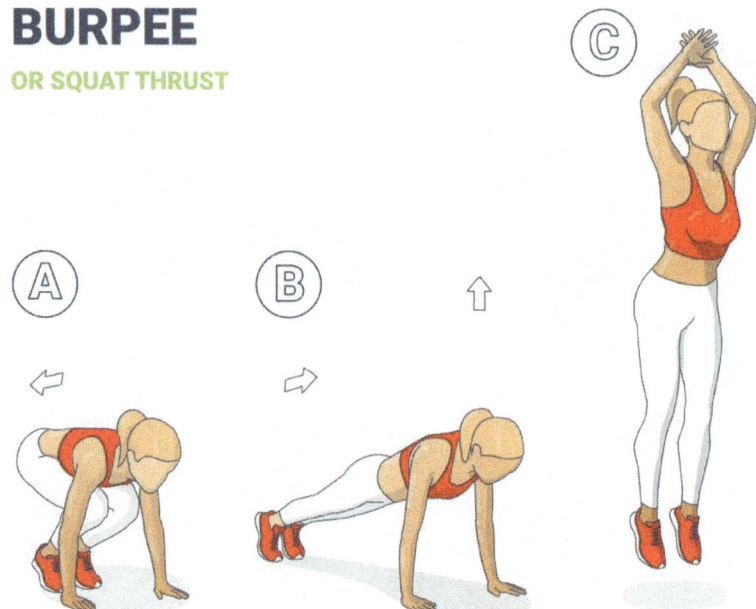

SQUAT JACKS

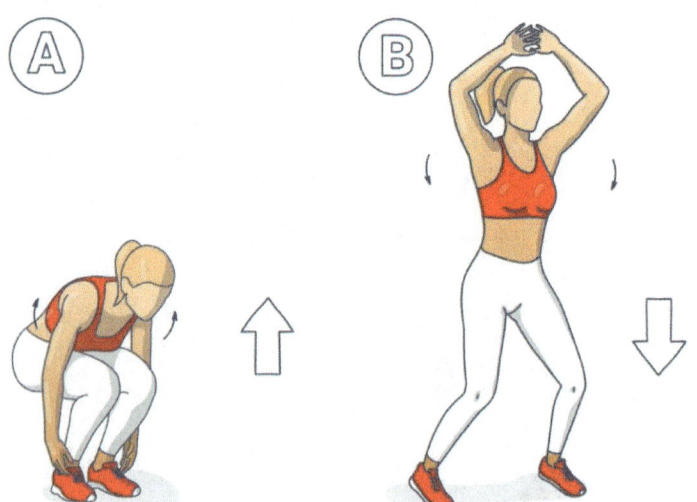

STANCE JACKS
VARIANT 1

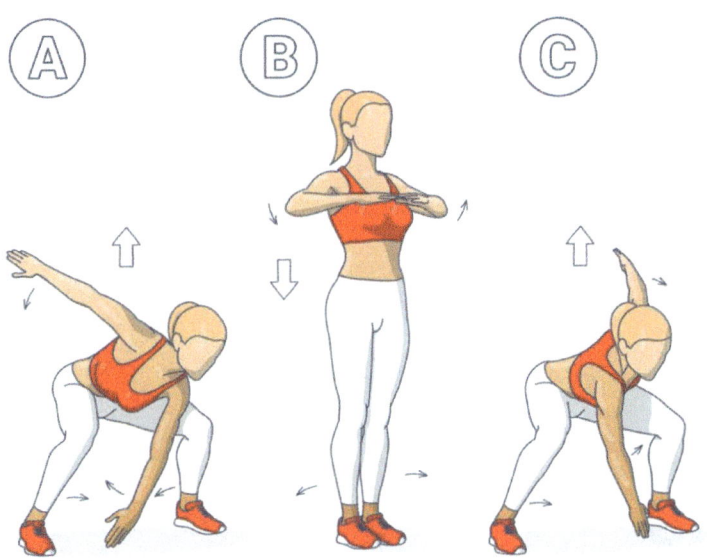

SNAP JUMPS

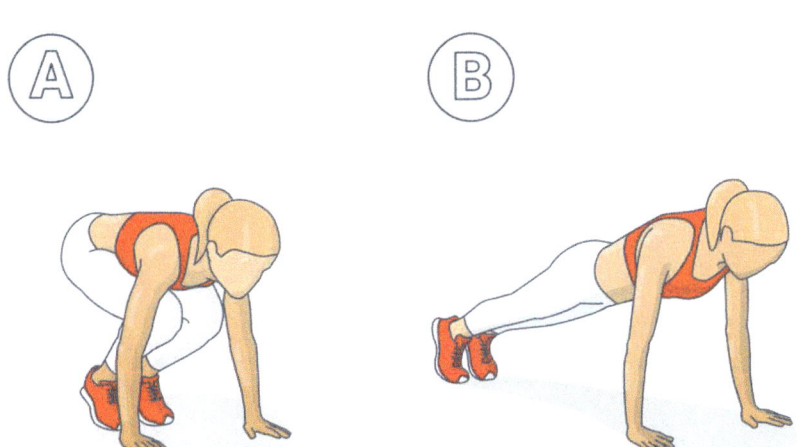

HIGH KNEES

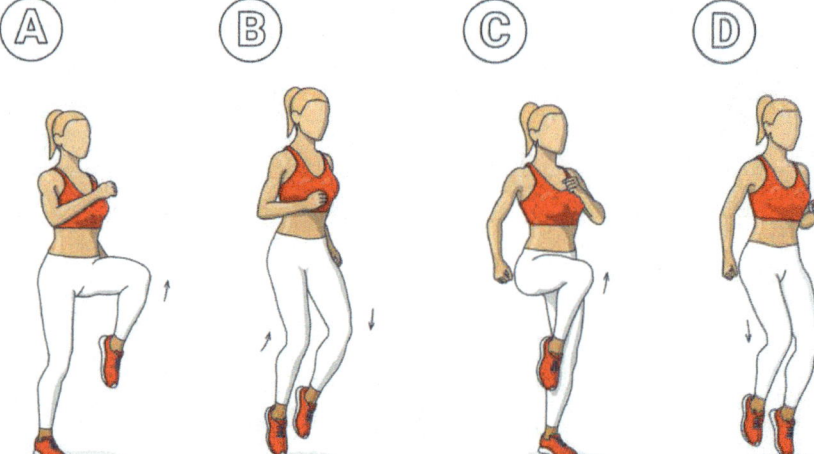

BUTT KICKS

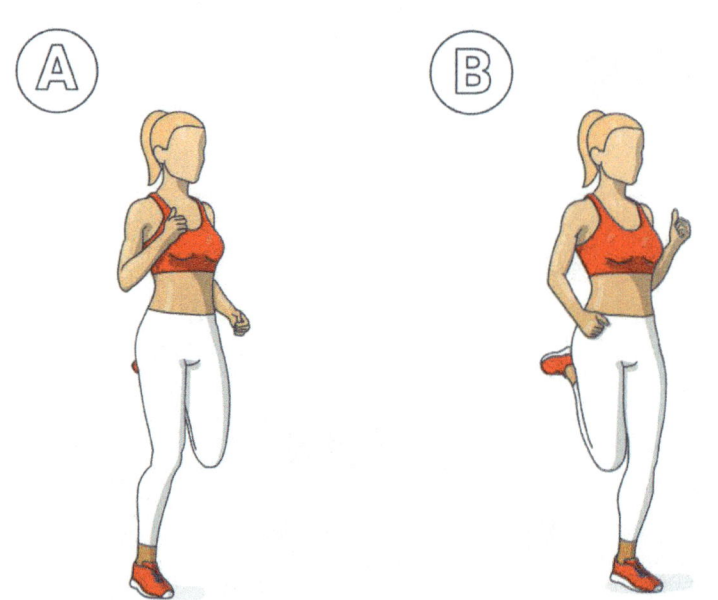

Core: Abs, glutes, and hips

SUMO GLUTE BRIDGE

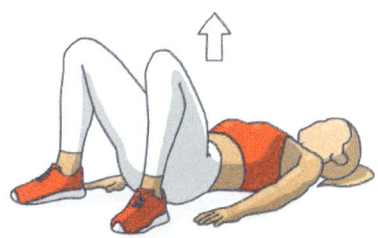
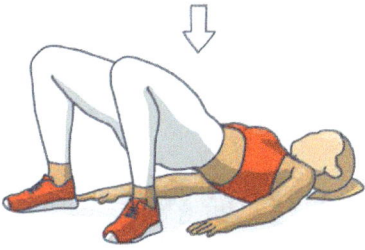

FULL PLANK **LOW PLANK**

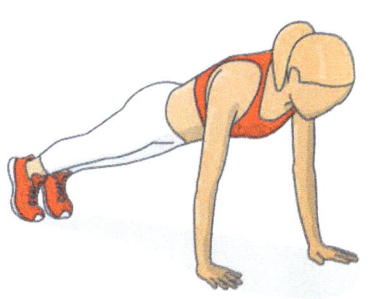
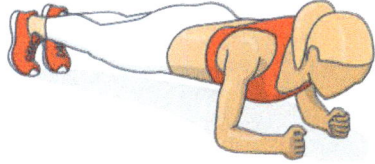

HIGH PLANK VARIATION WITH LEG RAISES
LEG RAISE PLANK

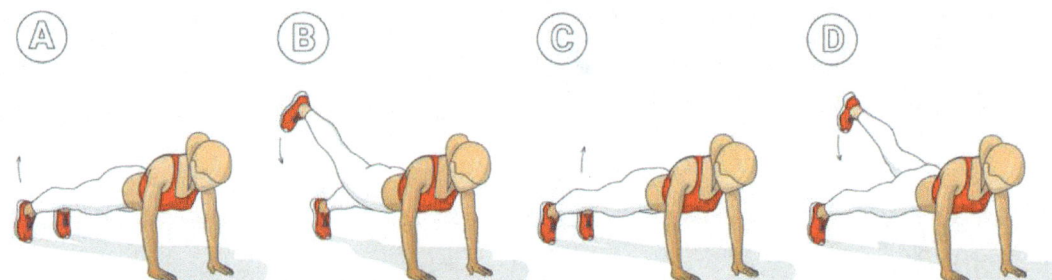

FIRE HYDRANT
WITH RESISTANCE BAND

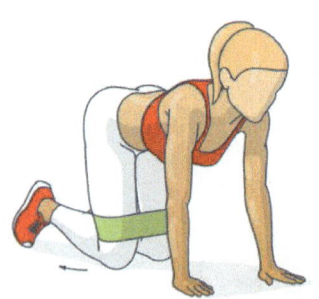
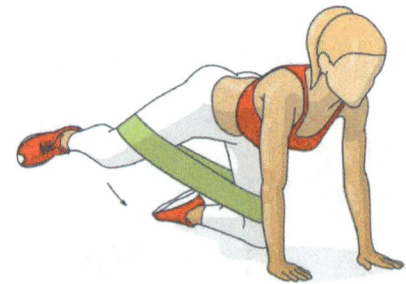

BIRD DOG
RIGHT HAND UP

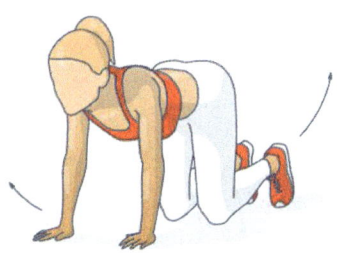 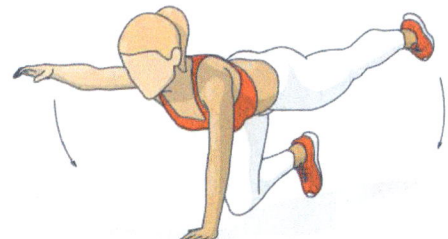

DONKEY KICK
WITH RESISTANCE BAND

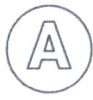

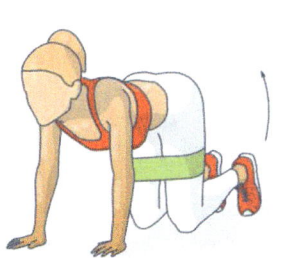 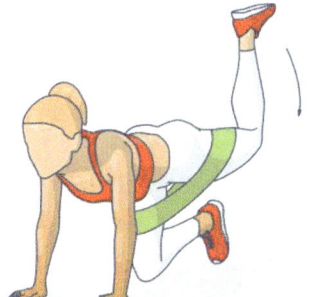

HIP THRUST

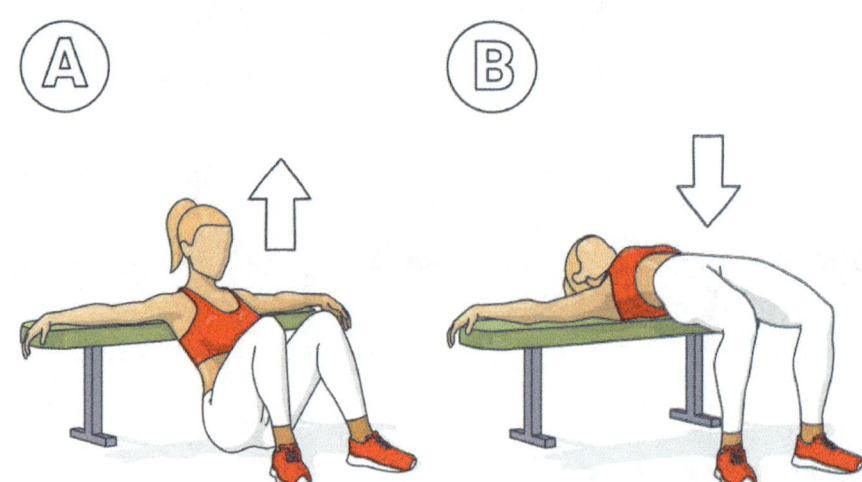

KNEE TO ELBOW
IN LOW PLANK

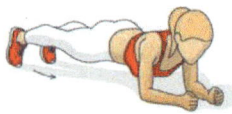 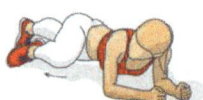 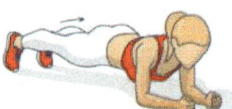 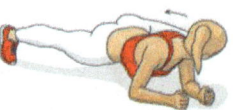

REVERSE CRUNCH
VARIATION #1

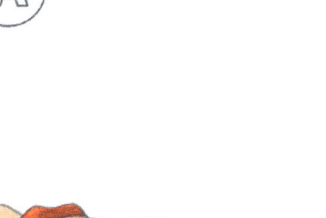
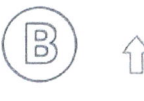
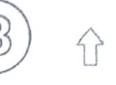
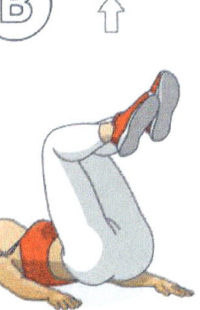
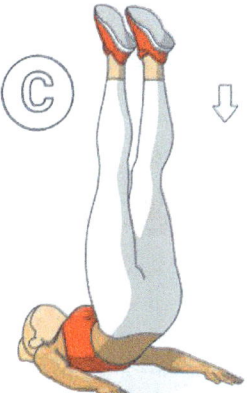

RUSSIAN TWIST
PRO VERSION

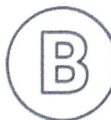
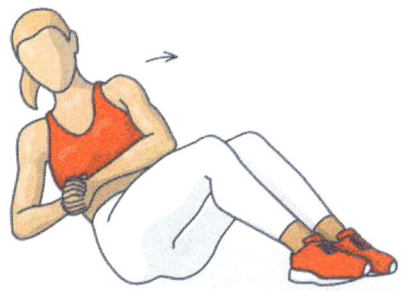
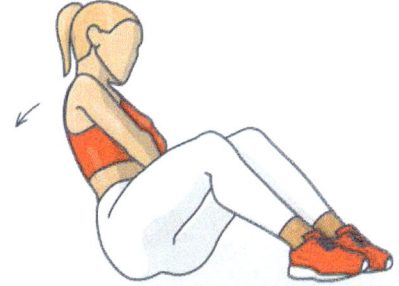

Quadriceps

AIR SQUATS

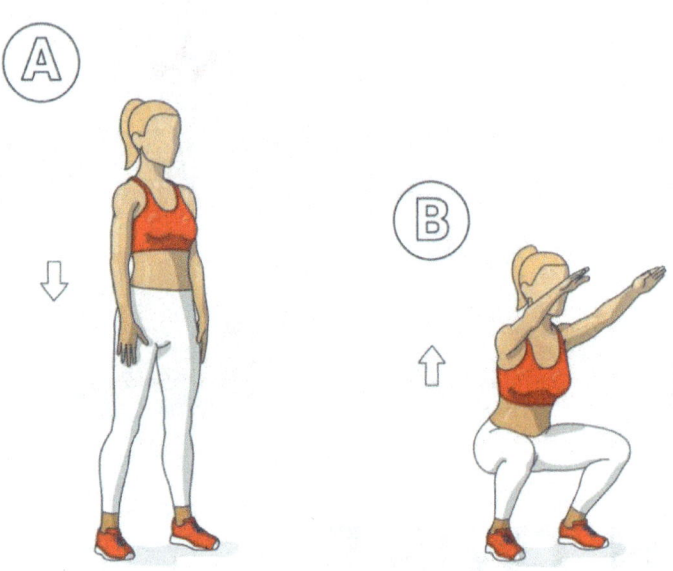

BELT KICKS

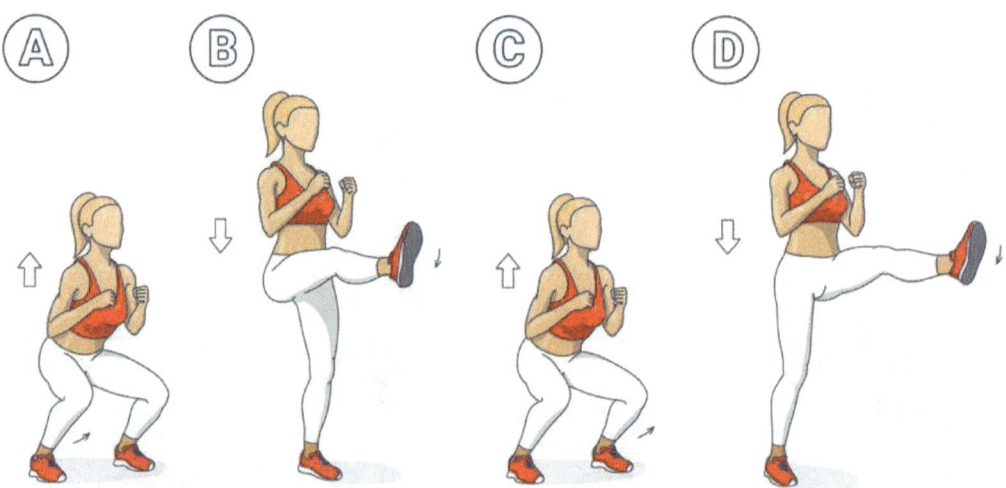

JUMP SQUATS
WITH RESISTANCE BAND

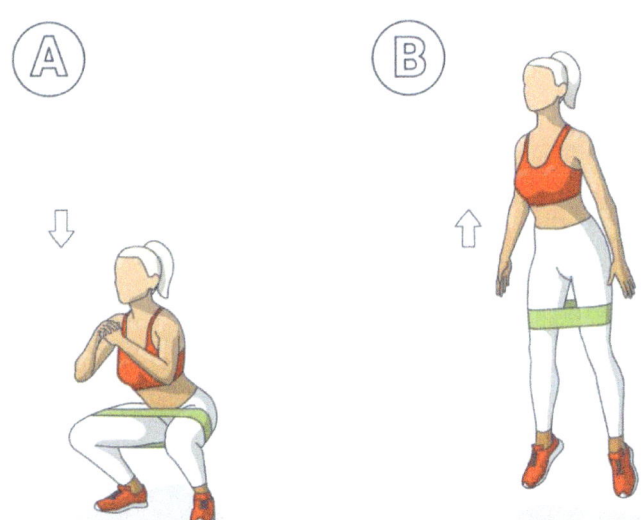

LATERAL STEPS & SQUATS
WITH RESISTANCE BAND

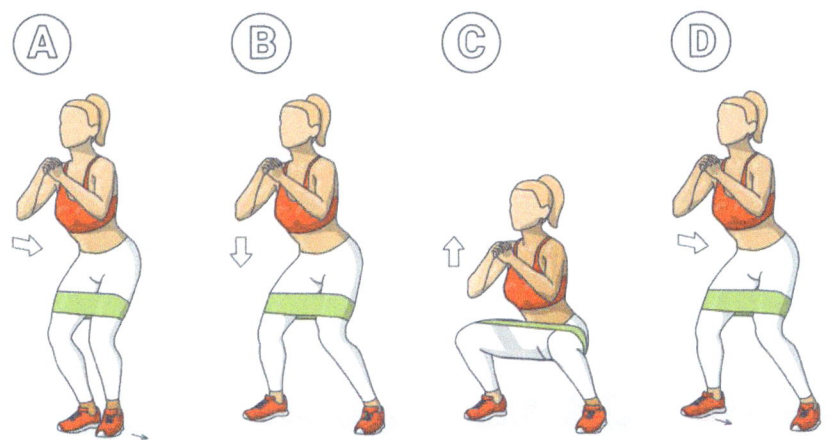

STEP UP

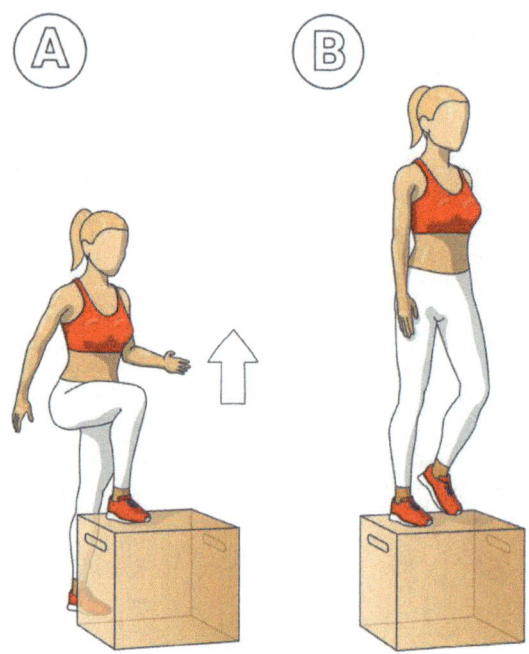

STEP-UP WITH A KNEE RAISE

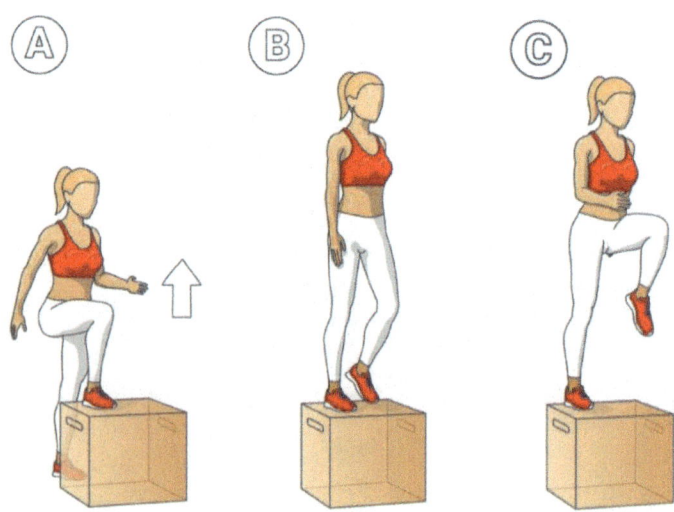

Hamstring

SWITCH KICKS
STANDING

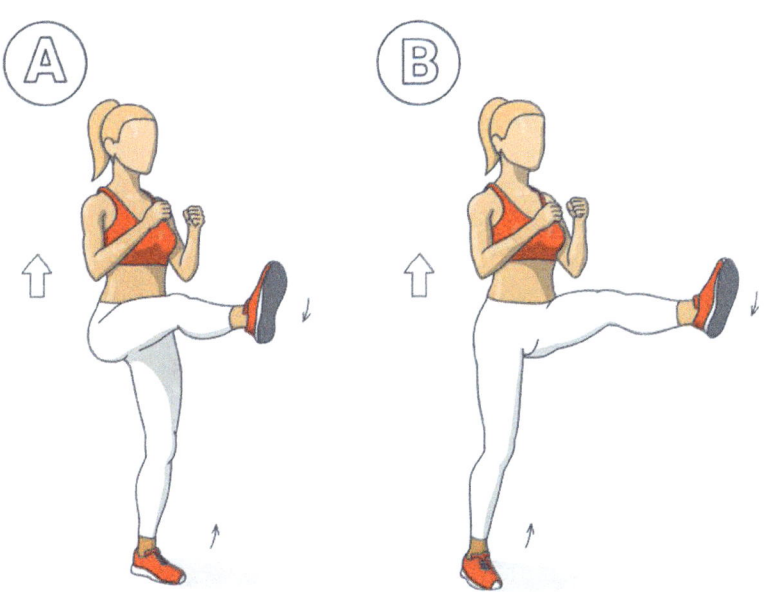

RAINBOW LEG LIFTS
WITH RESISTANCE BAND

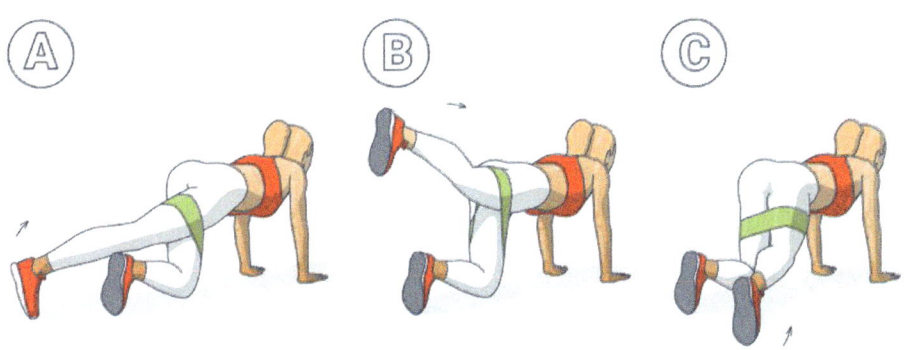

Abductor and adductor

SIDE PLANK LEG RAISE
BASIC VARIATION

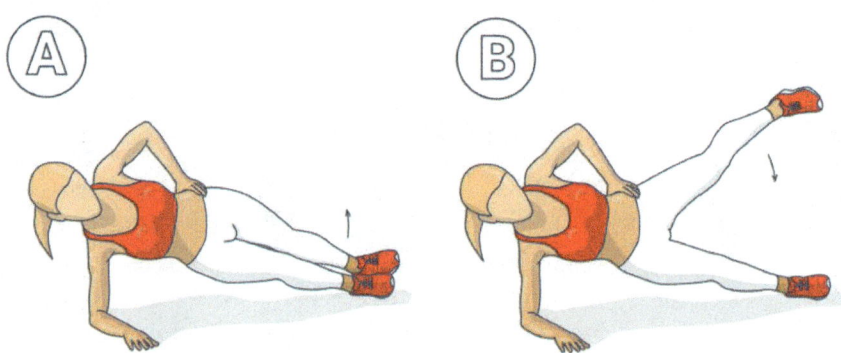

HIP ABDUCTION
WITH RESISTANCE BAND

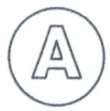
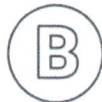

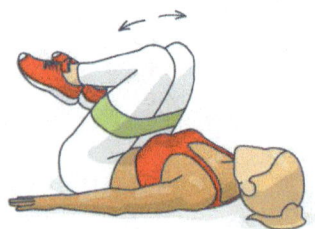
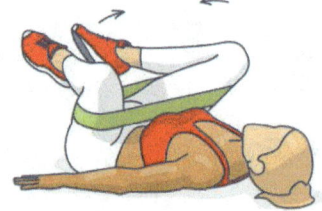

CLAMSHELL EXERCISE
WITH RESISTANCE BAND

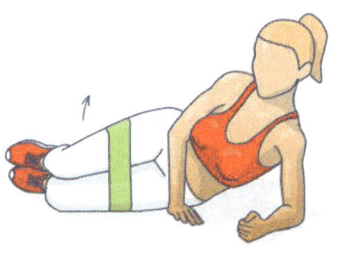
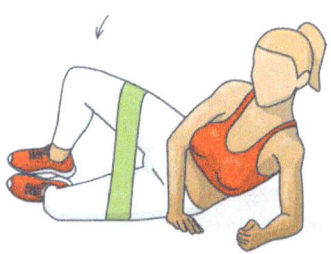

DUCK WALK
WITH RESISTANCE BAND

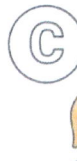
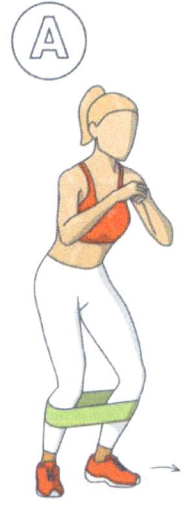
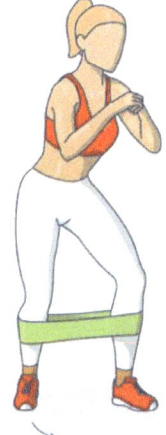
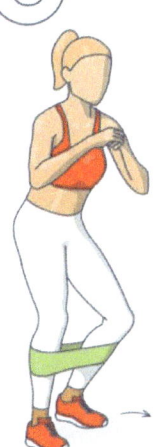

Back, chest and shoulder

KNEE PUSH-UPS

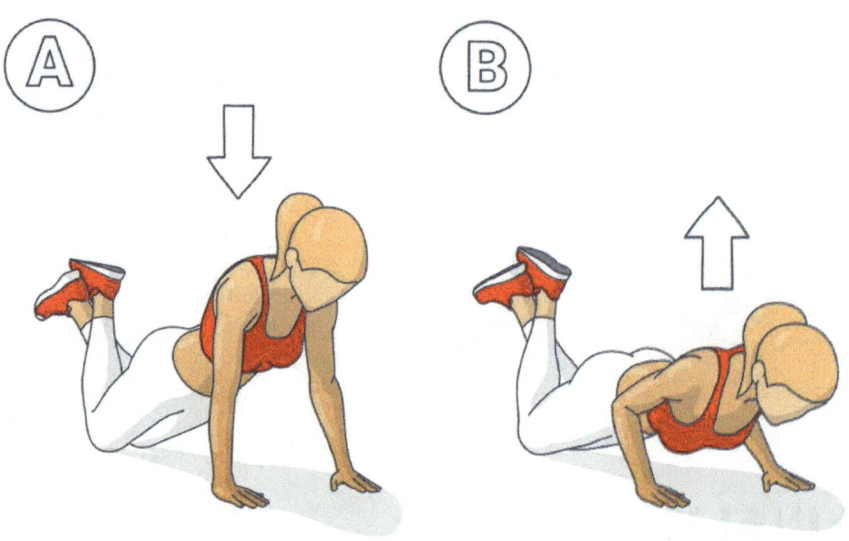

TRICEPS DIPS

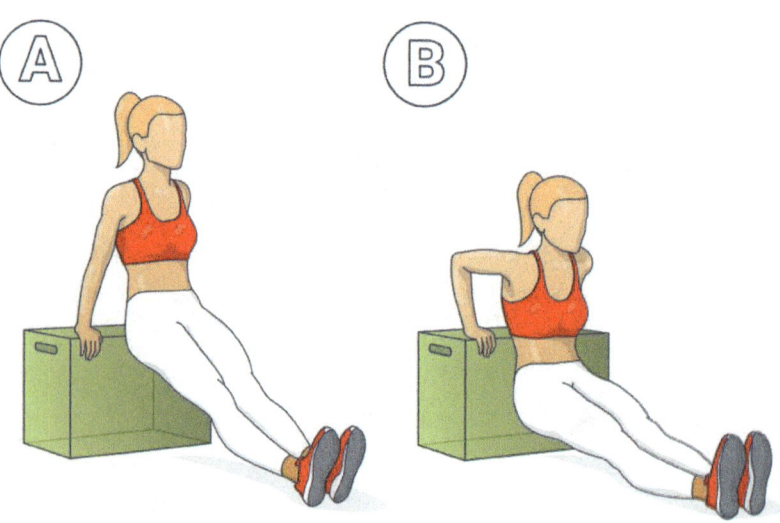

Made in the USA
Las Vegas, NV
09 August 2023

75876660R00066